Vegans Can't Eat Anything!

HEALTHY, ANIMAL-FRIENDLY COOKING

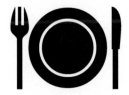

Catherine Greenall

Catherine Greenall

authorHOUSE®

AuthorHouse™ UK Ltd.
500 Avebury Boulevard
Central Milton Keynes, MK9 2BE
www.authorhouse.co.uk
Phone: 08001974150

First published by AuthorHouse   4/12/2010

ISBN: 978-1-4520-0370-2 (sc)

This book is printed on acid-free paper.

ALSO BY CATHERINE GREENALL

Vegans Can't Eat Anything! (Fully illustrated colour version)
Echoes
The Mersey Measure

**The cookbook you've been waiting for.
Easy to follow recipes for healthier
animal product-free food,
made from organic ingredients.**

The author recognises the challenges sometimes experienced in catering for vegans and so decided to share her own recipes. These include versions of regional dishes from her native Lancashire, dishes encountered in her travels and some she invented for herself. The titles of the book and chapters originate from what some restaurants actually said when asked for their vegan options. Whether you are vegan or vegetarian, or just want to eat more healthily for some meals, we are confident you will enjoy the dishes in this book

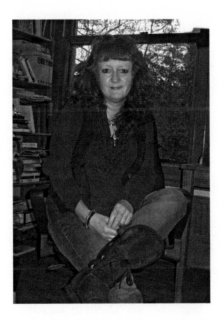

Acclaim for Vegans Can't Eat Anything!

Vegans can't eat anything - that is a common misconception. What is left? What on earth *can* you eat? The pictures look lovely! It's doing interesting things with fruit and vegetables...being creative and inventive with your food.

BBC Radio Manchester interview

So, as Cathy gave a short talk about the book, ignoring the friendly heckler asking if there was any bacon on the menu, I made my way over to the assorted tasters, tucking into mini roasted vegetable pizzas, nut rolls and Aloo Tikka Yums, which comprised tasty vegetables cooked with Indian spices, wrapped in filo pastry... one guest Molly, aged eleven, described it as the best pizza and tucked into another.. Cathy's book is packed with ideas for those who are interested in vegetarian and vegan dishes, but also for anyone who wants to boost their diet and their immune system, with some incredibly healthy recipes ideas.

Lancashire Life at the book launch for 'Vegans Can't Eat Anything!' Glasshouse Restaurant, Farmers Arms, Bispham.

The first thing that impressed me was the availability of the ingredients used. I found them to be easily accessible which is great as sometimes more obscure items are difficult to get hold of. Sometimes a recipe will be overlooked because one or two things are missing. The step by step instructions are also very well written and easy to follow, helping to avoid mistakes and disasters. The photos are very appetising and really make you want to make the food...the recipes will appeal not just to vegans/vegetarians but to all people who appreciate fine food. Altogether an entertaining and useful book that would be an asset to anyone's collection.

Mark Bateman, Vegan Society Merseyside

Catherine has written a cookbook that really challenges the notion that vegan cooking is dull. There are plenty of exciting recipes to make from simple teatime meals to gourmet evening meals to impress your guests. The recipes in the book are an interesting mix of international cuisine and also some traditional Lancashire dishes which is Catherine's home county. This cookbook contains recipes which will be enjoyed by vegans and non-vegans alike.

Wrexham Veggies (www.wrexhamveg.org)

The funny perceptions of non-Vegans are pretty laughable at times, but this great author, Catherine Greenall decided to take it an spin it into a fabulous book of vegan recipes.

easyvegetarianrecipes.spifty.com

This is a collection of Catherine's own recipes, and there is a good, well balanced selection with standard recipes such as Lentil Cottage Pie through to the more unusual and intriguing, including Beer Battered Beetroot!

Vegan Village

Dedication

This book is dedicated to Mum, Ann, my first teacher,
who inspired in me a love of good food and home cooking.

Acknowledgements

I would like to thank all those who have provided help, support and encouragement when I was writing this book.

In particular, I would like to thank the following:

To Alan for his constant encouragement, food testing and proof reading,

I want to thank Teresa, Judith and my Dad, Robert, for testing and tasting my recipes.

I would like to thank the Vegan Society for their encouragement and for allowing me to quote them as experts in the field.

I also really appreciate all those good friends who took a leap of faith and pre-ordered this book before even seeing it!

Contents

Illustrations

(Left to right)

Front Cover
Butternut Squash and Ginger Soup
Crispy Tempeh with Vegetables and Indonesian Satay Sauce
Normandy Apple Tart with Blackberry Sorbet

Back Cover
Bean, Olive and Salad Ciabatta
Halloween Squash Soup
Thai Puy Lentils
Black Peas
Nut Rolls
Roasted Vegetable Polenta Tart
Barbeque Aubergine Steaks, Crispy Leeks and Polenta Cakes
Mushroom and Nut Brandy Parcels with Rainbow Kale
Roasted Vegetable Pizza
Aubergine and Courgette Fritters with Chilli Dip
Beer-Battered Tempeh and Asparagus Tips
Bonfire Pie and Red Cabbage
Blueberry and Raspberry Cheesecake
Tipsy Blueberry Fool
Baked Polenta Custard Tart

Chapter 1: Why I Went Vegan

The title of this book is one of the first things that restaurants and hotels, not to mention friends and acquaintances, often say to me when I have imparted the shock news that I am vegan. This is usually just before they tell me that the menu does not contain anything for me.

Dining out is very challenging when you are vegan (or have any other dietary restriction, I would imagine). So what perverse chain of thought drove me to become such an awkward (and hated by chefs the world over) diner?

I first decided to become vegetarian in 1990. Cast your mind back to the second 'Summer of Love' in 1990. Agriculture Minister John Gummer was pictured cynically feeding his four-year-old daughter a burger to prove how safe British beef was in the middle of the 'mad cow disease' or BSE scare, which had been building up through the late 1980s. We didn't believe him then and a few years later, people in the UK were dying of CJD, the human form of BSE, for which there is no cure. The scandal had been covered up for years and was due to practices like feeding vegetarian animals the ground-up remains of other infected animals.

I was determined that contaminated meat products would not be on my menu. There were also many television programmes and news articles at the time, raising issues about exactly how the meat on our plates is produced. Animal welfare issues were being highlighted that I could not ignore, or be party to. I decided to go vegetarian.

I decided to only use Organic products whenever possible after becoming extremely concerned regarding revelations in the late 1990s on

Genetically Modified Food. A newspaper campaign publicised the fact that GM ingredients had been secretly introduced into our food, with no attempt to honestly label these.

Scientific research raising concerns about the effect of GM food on rats was stifled and one of the scientists concerned (Arpad Pusztai) vilified and dismissed. In addition, as a scientist myself, I was concerned about the impact on indigenous insect, plant and wildlife, as well as the effect on humans, of high levels of insect & weed killer used in growing foodstuffs. As a vegetarian, I was strongly opposed to the suggestion of the introduction of animal or human genes into food. For instance, experiments had been carried out to genetically modify strawberries with cold water fish genes to improve their shelf life. This was pretty abhorrent to a vegetarian (and to many others too).

GM foods proved to be a danger to human health in the USA, where 5000 victims of GM-adulterated L-tryptophan contracted an illness with flu-like symptoms, blistering of the skin, swollen livers and lungs and memory loss. L-tryptophan is one of the essential amino acids and is used to treat depression, insomnia and stress. This illness was diagnosed as eosinophilia myalagia syndrome (EMS) and was linked with the GM L-tryptophan. At least 37 of these victims died and more than 1500 were permanently disabled, until the US government officially stopped counting in 1991 and the product was withdrawn.

The benefits of this technology are not proven and the impact on human health has not been adequately assessed. The only sensible option seemed to be to buy organic produce, which is guaranteed free from genetic modification, pesticides and insecticides.

In 2001, there was a major outbreak of Foot and Mouth disease in the UK. This disease causes fever and blisters in cloven hoofed animals, but is not fatal and the animals would recover naturally. However, Government policy was to kill all herds where infected animals were identified. Around seven million animals were slaughtered and many farms went out of business. Dairy and meat cattle alike were killed in a distressing orgy of stinking, burning pyres that blackened our countryside. I did not wish to be a party to the productisation and casual disposal of animal life any longer and I went vegan.

Following a vegan diet is better not only for animals, but also for the environment and our health. The Vegan Society states[2] 'Every year a billion animals, most of them from factory farms, meet a cruel and early death to satisfy the demand for meat in the UK.'

Most of us recognise that we need to treat the environment with respect to preserve our resources for future generations. The Vegan Society states[2] 'Meat intensive diets contribute to worldwide environmental degradation – to global warming, deforestation, desertification, water pollution and the malnourishment of millions of people.'

There is a lot of concern in the UK about poor diet and obesity and links to illnesses, for example, heart disease, strokes and cancers. Witness the many television programmes about diet and its impact on good health and avoiding obesity. The Vegan Society states[2] that 'A well balanced wholefood vegan diet can improve your quality of life and decrease your chances of succumbing to many of the 'diseases of civilisation' – including heart disease, stroke, diabetes and some cancers.'

Recent concerns about climate change have highlighted the carbon emissions caused by transporting food over huge distances by road and air. In addition, the quality and nutritional value of fresh fruit and vegetables deteriorates with time after harvesting. It is therefore preferable to buy local produce when it is in season, where possible. You could even try growing your own!

So that is how I ended up being vegan and why I seek out organic, local produce wherever I can. There are lots of local vegetable growers and farmers markets these days and box schemes that will deliver fresh fruit and vegetables, as well as groceries. If you have to use the big supermarkets and we all need to sometimes, try to select local organic produce that hasn't been flown halfway round the world first.

I have tried to make my recipes healthy; they mostly use little fat, salt or sugar. I always try to prepare meals from the raw organic ingredients, rather than buying processed foods, although I occasionally use good quality pre-prepared ingredients. That way, I always know what is on my plate and the list does not sound like a chemistry experiment! Try to do the same where you can and I promise your food will taste better and you'll feel a lot healthier.

I hope you enjoy making at least some of these dishes as much as I have.

Catherine Greenall

Chapter 2:
'Sorry, the Vegetable Soup's got Cream in'
Appetising Starters & Snacks

Why do they do that? I mean, make a perfectly healthy fresh vegetable soup and then gunk it up with cream? Do even omnivores like their soup full of fat these days? It's the same when a veggie-sounding soup turns out to have a base of chicken stock. Save it for the chicken soup, chefs! Here are some you can make for yourself and it's dead easy.

Ideally you need a blender, unless you like your soup chunky. I like my soup to have quite a thick texture, but you can always add more stock if you like a thinner soup. I make no apologies for having so many soups in this section, as I think homemade soup is not only really comforting, it is also a really tasty way of contributing to your five-a-day portions of fruit and vegetables. So don't open that can, try making your own.

Avocado and Beetroot Open Sandwich

This makes a quick and colourful snack.

Serves 2

 4 slices wholemeal toast
 Salad leaves
 4 cherry tomatoes
 2 cooked beetroot
 2 spring onions
 2 avocados
 2 sticks celery
 Freshly ground black pepper

Dressing

 4 tablespoons wine vinegar
 1 tablespoon lemon juice
 1 tablespoon olive oil
 1 teaspoon brown sugar
 1 teaspoon mustard

1. Wash the salad leaves.
2. Cut the cherry tomatoes in half.
3. Slice the beetroot.
4. Cut the spring onions into 1 inch lengths.
5. Peel, stone and slice the avocados.
6. Cut the celery into thin slices.
7. Mix all the dressing ingredients in a screw top jar and shake well.
8. Cut the slices of toast in half diagonally and arrange on each plate.
9. Heap the salad leaves on the toast.
10. Arrange the sliced beetroot and cherry tomatoes on top.
11. Add the sliced avocado.
12. Scatter with the celery and spring onions.
13. Drizzle with the dressing, add black pepper to taste and serve.

Catherine Greenall

Avocado Bruschetta

Serves 2

1 ciabatta loaf
2-3 cloves garlic
4 large tomatoes
2-4 teaspoons of olive oil
1 handful of fresh (or 1 teaspoon of dried) basil
Black pepper
2 avocados
Juice of 1 lemon

1. Cut the ciabatta loaf in half lengthways, then cut each piece into two. Place cut side up on a baking tray.
2. Chop the garlic and slice the tomatoes.
3. Peel and chop the avocados. Place in a bowl and mix with the lemon juice.
4. Arrange the sliced tomatoes on the ciabatta and add the chopped garlic and black pepper to taste.
5. Drizzle with the olive oil and top with the chopped or dried basil.
6. Cook in a hot oven for 15 minutes, gas mark 4, electric 180C/ 350F.
7. Pile a spoonful of avocado on top of each piece of bruschetta and serve warm.

Bean and Mushroom Soup

Serves 2

1 onion
4 cloves garlic
6 -8 mushrooms
1 400g tin red kidney beans
2 teaspoons vegan bouillon
3/4 pint water
¼ pint white wine
1 teaspoon dried or fresh chives
Fresh basil to serve

1. Trim off stalk ends and chop the washed mushrooms.
2. Peel and chop the onion and garlic.
3. Place the chopped vegetables, kidney beans, water, wine, bouillon and chives in a large pan.
4. Bring to the boil and simmer for 20 minutes.
5. Blend the soup and serve topped with basil leaves, with crusty bread on the side.

Bean and Olive Salad Ciabatta

This sandwich is great for either your lunchbox,
picnic or as a filling snack.

Serves 2

1 ciabatta loaf

Filling

400g tin cooked kidney beans
10 olives
8 cherry tomatoes
Mixed leaf salad

Dressing

30ml balsamic vinegar
20ml sunflower oil
10ml olive oil
1 teaspoon French mustard
1 teaspoon brown sugar
Black pepper
Chopped garlic

1. Place the dressing ingredients in a screw top jar and shake well.
2. Place the kidney beans, olives and cherry tomatoes in a bowl.
3. Add the dressing and marinate in the refrigerator for 1 hour.
4. Wrap the ciabatta in foil and warm in the oven for 10 minutes; gas mark 4, electric 180C/ 350F.
5. Split the ciabatta lengthways, then cut each length into two pieces.
6. Arrange two pieces of bread on each plate and top with washed salad leaves.
7. Add the marinated bean and olive mixture on top and serve.

(See back cover for photograph)

Black Peas

This is a speciality of the Lancashire area where I grew up. The old fashioned fairgrounds and fêtes always had a black pea stall, where the peas were ladled out in a thick soup with a dash of vinegar and pepper.

Serves 4

1 400g bag of dried black peas (sometimes known as pigeon peas)
0.5 pint water
1 teaspoons vegan bouillon
Balsamic vinegar
Freshly ground black pepper

1. Soak the black peas in double the volume of water overnight.
2. Rinse the peas in cold water several times.
3. Add the water and bouillon.
4. Bring to the boil and simmer for 2-3 hours.
5. Serve peas with some of the liquid in a bowl.
6. Add a slug of balsamic vinegar and some freshly ground black pepper to each bowl and serve hot.

(See back cover for photograph)

Butternut Squash and Ginger Soup

Try this starter for a special occasion.

Serves 2

> 1 peeled and de-seeded butternut squash
> 1 onion
> 2-3 cloves garlic
> 2 small – medium potatoes
> 2 teaspoons of olive oil
> 1 pint water
> 2 teaspoons organic vegan bouillon
> 2 teaspoons ground ginger or chopped root ginger

Freshly ground black pepper and soya yoghurt to finish

1. Peel and chop the butternut squash, removing the seeds. Chop the onion, garlic and potatoes.
2. Fry the chopped vegetables in the olive oil for a few minutes, stirring occasionally.
3. Add the water, ginger and organic vegan bouillon (or other vegetable stock).
4. Bring to the boil; then simmer for around 20-30 minutes until the vegetables are cooked.
5. Blend all the liquid and serve, topped with a swirl of soya yoghurt and freshly ground black pepper.

(See front cover for photograph)

Celeriac, Carrot and Coconut Soup

This is a creamy soup, made with a delicious-tasting, but much-neglected vegetable.

Serves 2

1 onion
2 cloves garlic
1 celeriac
2 carrots
2 teaspoons olive oil
2 teaspoons coriander
0.5 teaspoon turmeric
1 pint of water
2 teaspoons vegan bouillon
50g slice creamed coconut
2 tablespoons lime juice
Freshly chopped parsley for garnish

1. Peel and chop the onion, garlic, celeriac and carrots.
2. Fry the onion and garlic in the oil in a large pan for 2 minutes. Add the coriander and turmeric and stir fry for 1 minute.
3. Add water, the vegan bouillon, chopped celeriac and carrot.
4. Add the lime juice and creamed coconut and mix well.
5. Bring to the boil; then simmer for around 20-30 minutes until vegetables are cooked.
6. Blend all the liquid and serve topped with the parsley.

Celeriac, Courgette and Mint Soup

Serves 2

> 1 onion
> 2 cloves garlic
> 1 celeriac
> 2 courgettes
> 1 pint of water
> 2 teaspoons vegan bouillon
> Handful of mint leaves
> Freshly chopped mint for garnish

1. Peel and chop the onion, garlic, celeriac and courgettes into a large saucepan.
2. Add water, the vegan bouillon and the chopped handful of mint.
3. Bring to the boil; then simmer for around 20-30 minutes until vegetables are cooked.
4. Blend all the liquid and serve topped with the chopped mint.

Chilli Bean Soup

If you like your soup hot, this one's just for you!

Serves 2

> 1 onion
> 3 cloves garlic
> 6 chillies
> 1 400g tin tomatoes
> 1 400g tin red kidney beans
> 2 teaspoons vegan bouillon
> 0.5 pint water
> 2 tablespoons tomato puree

1. Chop the onion, garlic and chillies.
2. Place the chopped vegetables and all other ingredients in a large pan.
3. Bring to the boil and simmer for 20 minutes.
4. Blend the soup, serve and fill your iced water glass!

Garlic Roasted Baby Aubergine Salad

Serves 2

2 baby aubergines
1 tablespoon olive oil
2 cloves garlic
Salad to serve

Dressing

30ml balsamic vinegar
20ml sunflower oil
30ml olive oil
1 teaspoon French mustard
1 teaspoon brown sugar
Black pepper

1. Wash the aubergines and slice into two or three thick pieces lengthways.
2. Place the aubergine slices in a baking tray, drizzle with the olive oil and add chopped garlic. Bake in the oven for 30 minutes; gas mark 4, electric 180C/ 350F.
3. Place the dressing ingredients in a screw top jar and shake well.
4. Arrange the salad on serving dishes and top with the roasted aubergine.
5. Drizzle with the dressing and serve.

Halloween Squash Soup

Have some fun whilst making this spicy soup for Halloween!

Serves 2

1 medium – large squash
1 onion
2 cloves garlic
2 teaspoons olive oil
2 carrots
2 potatoes
2 teaspoons curry powder
0.5 teaspoon turmeric
1 pint of water
50g slice creamed coconut
2 teaspoons vegan bouillon
1 teaspoon dried (or a handful of fresh) coriander leaves to decorate

1. Cut a lid from the top of the squash and scoop out the flesh from inside and reserve flesh in a bowl. Remove any seeds.
2. You can now cut eye nose and mouth holes in the squash shell for a Halloween lantern. Place a tea light inside and replace the lid.
3. Chop the onion, garlic, squash flesh, carrots and potatoes.
4. Fry the onion and garlic in the oil in a large pan for 2 minutes. Add the curry powder and turmeric and stir fry for 1 minute.
5. Add water, the vegan bouillon, squash flesh, carrots, potatoes and creamed coconut.
6. Bring to the boil; then simmer for around 20-30 minutes until vegetables are cooked.
7. Blend all the liquid and serve topped with the coriander leaves. Happy Halloween!

(See back cover for photograph)

Hummus & Sun Dried Tomato on Ciabatta

Hummus contains chick peas, which are a great source of protein.

Serves 2

 1 200g tub of hummus
 2 ciabatta rolls
 8 sun-dried tomatoes
 6 cherry tomatoes
 2 sticks celery
 Mixed salad leaves

Dressing

 30ml balsamic vinegar
 30ml olive oil
 1 teaspoon French mustard
 1 teaspoon brown sugar
 Black pepper

1. Slice the sun-dried tomatoes into strips.
2. Mix the dressing ingredients in a screw top jar, shake well and keep chilled.
3. Wash the cherry tomatoes and cut into halves.
4. Wash the salad leaves and trimmed celery sticks and drain on kitchen paper.
5. Finely slice the celery.
6. Cut the ciabatta rolls in half and toast.
7. Place a thick layer of hummus on each half of ciabatta roll and arrange on plates.
8. Add the sun-dried tomato strips on top.
9. Add the salad leaves, celery and cherry tomatoes.
10. Drizzle with the dressing and serve.

Leek, Sweet Potato & Mint Soup

This is a warming, nutritious soup.

Serves 2

2-3 leeks
1-2 sweet potatoes
2 teaspoons dried mint (or mint in vinegar from a jar)
2 teaspoons vegan bouillon
1 pint water
1 slice of bread
2 teaspoons sunflower oil

1. Top and tail the leeks and remove the outer leaves.
2. Cut each leek lengthways, then slice each half of leek into thin semicircles. Place the sliced leek into a colander and wash thoroughly with cold water, separating the layers to ensure removal of trapped soil.
3. Peel and chop the sweet potatoes.
4. Place the leeks, sweet potatoes, mint, bouillon and water in a large pan.
5. Bring to the boil and simmer for 30 minutes.
6. Meanwhile, chop the bread into small squares. Heat the sunflower oil in a small frying pan and fry the bread croutons until crisp and brown.
7. Blend the soup and serve topped with the croutons.

Minted Pea Soup

This is a tasty, colourful protein and iron-rich soup.

Serves 2

- 1 onion
- 1 cup split peas
- 1 pint water
- 2 teaspoons vegan bouillon
- 1 teaspoon dried (or a handful of fresh) mint
- 2 sun dried tomatoes

1. Chop the onion into a large pan and add all of the other ingredients, except for the sun dried tomatoes.
2. Bring to the boil; then simmer for an hour.
3. Cut the sun dried tomatoes into thin strips.
4. Blend all the liquid and serve, topped with the sun dried tomatoes.

Catherine Greenall

Mung Dal, Lime and Coconut Soup

Mung, or moong, dal is an Indian yellow bean made from
hulled, split green mung beans. Mung dal is low in fat and
a good source of vitamins, protein and minerals.

Serves 2

 1 onion
 2-3 cloves garlic
 1 cup mung dhal
 1 pint water
 2 teaspoons vegan bouillon
 2 teaspoons chopped lemongrass
 2 tablespoons lime juice
 50g slice creamed coconut
 Rocket, watercress and spinach (or other mixed leaves) to serve

1. Chop the onion and garlic.
2. Rinse the mung dhal in cold water several times.
3. Add the onion, garlic, mung dhal, water, bouillon, lemongrass, lime juice and creamed coconut to a large pan.
4. Bring to the boil and simmer for 50 minutes.
5. Serve topped with a handful of the washed mixed leaves.

Mushroom and White Wine Soup

Serves 2

2 cloves garlic
8-10 mushrooms
2 teaspoons olive oil
150ml white wine
300ml of water
2 teaspoons vegan bouillon
1 teaspoon of mint leaves in vinegar
2 medium potatoes
4 leaves seasonal greens (I used green cabbage here)
1 spring onion (green stem only)

1. Peel and chop the garlic and mushrooms and place in a large saucepan.
2. Add the olive oil and fry stirring for a few minutes.
3. Add the white wine, water, the vegan bouillon and the mint.
4. Add the peeled, chopped potatoes and shredded greens.
5. Boil then simmer for 20-30 minutes, until vegetables are cooked.
6. Trim the washed spring onion greens and cut into thin shreds.
7. Blend all the liquid and serve, topped with the shredded spring onion.

Parsnip & Sweetcorn Soup

Parsnips are packed with vitamins and sweetcorn
contains stress-busting vitamins.

Serves 2

1 onion
2 cloves garlic
2 parsnips
1 carrot
1 pint water
2 cups sweetcorn
1 teaspoon dried parsley
2 teaspoons vegan bouillon

1. Chop the onion, garlic, parsnips and carrot into a large saucepan.
2. Add the water, sweetcorn, parsley and bouillon and bring to the boil.
3. Simmer for 30 minutes and serve.

Potato and Balsamic Mint Soup

This is a lovely, fresh-tasting soup for a summer's day.

Serves 2

3 tablespoons balsamic vinegar
1 teaspoon brown sugar
Black pepper
1 handful of mint leaves
2 large potatoes
1 onion
2 teaspoons vegan bouillon
Mint leaves for garnish

1. Mix the balsamic vinegar with the brown sugar and add a sprinkling of black pepper.
2. Marinate the chopped mint leaves in the balsamic marinade for 1 hour.
3. Chop the potato and onion and place in a large saucepan. Add 1 pint of water, the marinated balsamic mint and the vegan bouillon. Bring to the boil.
4. Simmer for 20-30 minutes until cooked.
5. Blend the soup and serve hot or cold, topped with chopped mint.

Spicy Butternut Squash Soup

This is a spicy soup for an autumn day.

Serves 2

1 onion
2-3 cloves garlic
2 teaspoons of olive oil
1 teaspoon of curry powder
Fresh coriander leaves or 1 teaspoon of coriander
Half a teaspoon of turmeric
1 pint water
2 teaspoons organic vegan bouillon
1 peeled and de-seeded butternut squash
Fresh coriander leaves to finish

1. Fry chopped onion and garlic in olive oil for a few minutes.
2. Add curry powder, coriander and turmeric and stir fry for a few seconds.
3. Add the water and organic vegan bouillon (or other vegetable stock).
4. Add butternut squash, chopped into small cubes.
5. Bring to the boil; then simmer for around 20-30 minutes until vegetables are cooked.
6. Blend all the liquid and serve, topped with chopped coriander.

Spicy Lentil Soup

Serves 2

- 1 onion
- 2-3 cloves garlic
- 2 teaspoons olive oil
- 1 teaspoon curry powder
- 2 teaspoons coriander
- 2 carrots
- 1 sweet potato
- 1 pint water
- 2 teaspoons vegan bouillon
- 2 cups split red lentils
- 50g slice creamed coconut

1. Chop the onion and garlic and fry in the olive oil in a saucepan for a few minutes.
2. Add the curry powder and coriander. Fry with stirring for a few seconds.
3. Chop the carrots and sweet potato and add to the pan.
4. Add the water, bouillon, lentils and creamed coconut.
5. Bring to the boil and simmer for 50 minutes.
6. Blend and serve.

Spicy Sweet Potato and Red Pepper Soup

This is a rich, colourful soup for a special occasion.

Serves 2

1 onion
2-3 cloves garlic
2 teaspoons of olive oil
1 teaspoon of curry powder
1 teaspoon of coriander
1 quarter teaspoon of turmeric
1 pint water
2 teaspoons vegan bouillon
2 small (or 1 large) peeled, chopped sweet potatoes
1 chopped red pepper
0.5 aubergine
Olive oil to roast

1. Fry chopped onion and garlic in olive oil for a few minutes.
2. Add curry powder, coriander and turmeric and stir fry for a few seconds.
3. Add water, vegan bouillon (or other vegetable stock), chopped sweet potatoes and chopped red pepper.
4. Bring to the boil; then simmer for around 20-30 minutes until vegetables are cooked.
5. Meanwhile, slice the aubergine fairly thinly and place slices in a baking tray coated with olive oil. Turn slices to
6. coat with the oil. Roast in a hot oven for 30 minutes, gas mark 4, electric 180C/ 350F.
7. Blend all the liquid. Serve the soup topped with slices of roasted aubergine.

Sweet Potato, Courgette & Coriander Soup

This is one of my favourite soups.

Serves 2

1 onion
2-3 cloves garlic
2 teaspoons of olive oil
1 teaspoon of cumin
1 pint water
2 teaspoons vegan bouillon
2 small (or 1 large) chopped sweet potatoes
2 sliced courgettes
Fresh coriander (or 2 teaspoons dried coriander)

1. Fry chopped onion and garlic in olive oil for a few minutes.
2. Add cumin and fry for a few seconds.
3. Add water, vegan bouillon (or other vegetable stock), chopped sweet potatoes, sliced courgettes and fresh or dried coriander.
4. Bring to the boil; then simmer for around 20-30 minutes until vegetables are cooked.
5. Blend all the liquid and serve soup topped with chopped fresh coriander.

Tempeh & Sweetcorn Soup

Tempeh is made from fermented soya beans and contains
protein. Sweetcorn contains stress-busting vitamins.

Serves 2

> 3 sticks tempeh
> 1 teaspoon dried ginger
> 2 tablespoons sherry
> 2 tablespoons flour
> 1 pint water
> 2 cups sweetcorn
> 2 teaspoons vegan bouillon
> 1 tablespoon soy sauce

1. Cut the tempeh into strips and mix with the ginger and sherry in a bowl.
2. Mix the flour with a small amount of cold water until smooth.
3. Place the water, sweetcorn and bouillon into a large pan and boil for 5 minutes.
4. Add the tempeh mixture and bring back to the boil.
5. Add the blended flour and water and the soy sauce.
6. Bring back to the boil; then simmer for a few minutes until the soup thickens.
7. Serve.

Thai Beancurd and Vegetable Soup (Tom Yum Tofu)

This is my favourite Thai soup.

Serves 2

1 250g pack beancurd (tofu)
1 red pepper
1 carrot
6 leaves winter green cabbage
1 onion
3 cloves garlic
2 teaspoons of olive oil
1 teaspoon curry powder
2 teaspoons chilli powder or 6 chopped fresh chillies
0.5 teaspoon turmeric
50g slice of creamed coconut
Juice of 1 lime
2 teaspoons Thai Holy Basil
2 teaspoons vegan organic bouillon

1. Cut the tofu lengthways into slices, then cut each slice into about 3cm strips.
2. Finely slice the red pepper and carrot.
3. Cut the cabbage into thin strips.
4. Chop the onion and garlic.
5. Heat the olive oil in a large pan, add the onions and garlic and stir fry for 2 minutes.
6. Add the curry powder, chilli powder or fresh chillies and turmeric. Fry stirring regularly for a minute
7. Add 1 pint water, coconut and the bouillon, and stir well, bring to the boil.
8. Add the red pepper, carrot, cabbage, tofu, Thai Holy Basil and lime juice. Mix well and simmer for 10-15 minutes.

Thai Puy Lentils

This can be served alone as a snack or with boiled
rice or rice noodles as a main course.

Serves 2

1 onion
2-3 cloves garlic
2 teaspoons olive oil
2 red chillies
1 teaspoon curry powder
2 teaspoons coriander
0.5 teaspoon turmeric
400ml can of coconut milk
0.5 pint water
2 teaspoons vegan bouillon
2 cups puy lentils
1 teaspoon chopped lemongrass
1 handful of fresh basil

1. Chop the onion and garlic and fry in the olive oil in a saucepan for a few minutes.
2. Chop the chillies finely.
3. Add the curry powder, coriander, turmeric and chopped chillies. Fry with stirring for a few seconds.
4. Add the coconut milk and mix thoroughly.
5. Add the water, bouillon, lentils and lemongrass.
6. Bring to the boil and simmer for 50 minutes.
7. Serve topped with the basil leaves.

(See back cover for photograph)

Tomato and Basil Soup

This is a light, Italian –style soup.

Serves 2

1 onion
2-3 sticks celery
2-3 cloves garlic
2 teaspoons of olive oil
Fresh basil leaves or 1 teaspoon of dried basil
1 400g tin of tomatoes
0.5 pint water
2 teaspoons vegan bouillon
4 tablespoons tomato puree
Chopped basil to garnish

1. Chop the onion, celery and garlic and place into a large pan.
2. Add olive oil, fresh or dried basil and the tinned tomatoes.
3. Add water, vegan bouillon (or other vegetable stock) and tomato puree.
4. Bring to the boil; then simmer for around 20-30 minutes until vegetables are cooked.
5. Blend all the liquid and serve soup, topped with chopped basil.

Tomato Chilli and Split Pea Soup

Serves 2

 1 onion
 2-3 cloves garlic
 2 teaspoons olive oil
 2 teaspoons coriander
 1 400g tin tomatoes
 0.5 pint water
 2 teaspoons vegan bouillon
 1 cup split yellow peas
 3 chopped chillies

1. Chop the onion and garlic and fry in the olive oil in a saucepan for a few minutes.
2. Add the coriander. Fry with stirring for a few seconds.
3. Add the tomatoes, water, bouillon and split peas.
4. Chop the chillies and add to the pan.
5. Bring to the boil and simmer for 2 hours.
6. Blend and serve.

Turnip and Sweetcorn Soup

These ingredients are full of vitamins and produce a sunny, yellow soup.

Serves 2

1 onion
1 turnip
¾ pint of water
¼ pint soya milk
2 teaspoons vegan bouillon
1 teaspoon dried or fresh chives
1 cup sweetcorn
Fresh basil leaves for garnish

1. Peel and chop the onion and turnip into a large saucepan.
2. Add water, chives and the vegan bouillon.
3. Bring to the boil; then simmer for 20 minutes.
4. Add sweetcorn and soya milk.
5. Bring back to the boil and simmer for 10 minutes.
6. Blend all the liquid and serve topped with the basil leaves.

Catherine Greenall

Turnip, Parsnip and Coriander Soup

Serves 2

    1 onion
    2 cloves garlic
    1 turnip
    1 large or 2 small parsnips
    2 teaspoons olive oil
    2 teaspoons coriander
    1 pint of water
    2 teaspoons vegan bouillon
    Freshly chopped mint for garnish

1. Peel and chop the onion, garlic, turnip and parsnips into a large saucepan.
2. Add the olive oil and fry for a few minutes.
3. Add the coriander and fry stirring for 1 minute.
4. Add water and the vegan bouillon.
5. Bring to the boil; then simmer for around 30 minutes until vegetables are cooked.
6. Blend all the liquid and serve topped with the chopped mint.

Warm Asparagus and Brazil Nut Salad

Asparagus contains no fat and is a good source of vitamins and minerals.

Serves 2

Salad

    12 sticks asparagus
    1 red onion
    1 cooked cold beetroot
    1 large carrot
    Salad leaves
    12 Brazil nuts
    2 sticks celery
    Black pepper

Balsamic Dressing

    3 tablespoons of balsamic vinegar
    1 teaspoon brown sugar
    I tablespoon of olive oil

1. Trim hard ends of stalk from asparagus and then steam whole for 10-15 minutes. Set aside to cool slightly.
2. Chop the red onion into a bowl and grate the carrot into a separate bowl.
3. Slice the beetroot and celery thinly.
4. Mix the dressing ingredients in a screw-top jar and shake well.
5. Place washed salad leaves on a plate, arrange sliced celery, beetroot slices and grated carrot on the plate.
6. Arrange warm asparagus on top of each salad. Decorate with chopped red onion and Brazil nuts.
7. Pour over the dressing and add black pepper to taste.

Winter Vegetable Soup

This is a hearty soup for a cold day.

Serves 2

2 carrots
6 winter cabbage leaves
1 large potato
1 onion
1 pint of water
2 teaspoons vegan bouillon
1 teaspoon dried (or a handful of fresh) parsley

1. Chop the carrots, cabbage, potato and onion into a large pan.
2. Add water, the vegan bouillon and parsley.
3. Bring to the boil; then simmer for around 20-30 minutes until vegetables are cooked.
4. Blend all the liquid and serve.

Chapter 3:
'We Could Do You a Plain Salad?'
Nourishing Main Courses

When you go out to a restaurant with friends and realise there is nothing on the menu that you can eat, even if you ask them to omit most of the listed ingredients and then they say that they could make you a plain salad, your heart just sinks. OK, salads are great in the summer, but on a cold wintry day you just want to eat something hot and tasty, just like everyone else. Well, try these out.

Aloo Tikka Yums with Yoghurt Dip

This dish is simply delicious! Vegetables are cooked with Indian spices, wrapped in filo pastry and served with a garlicky yoghurt dip. Great with salad and potato wedges.

Makes 10-12

Yums

2 onions
2 cloves garlic
2 teaspoons olive oil
2 teaspoons cumin
1 teaspoon coriander
½ pint water
1 teaspoon vegan bouillon
2 carrots
2 sweet potatoes
2 potatoes
1 250g pack filo pastry

Dip

250ml soya yoghurt
1 piece cucumber - about 4"
1 clove garlic
1 teaspoon mint in vinegar

Yums

1. Peel and chop the onions and garlic. Fry in the olive oil in a saucepan for 5 minutes.
2. Add cumin and coriander and continue to fry for a couple of minutes.
3. Add water and bouillon and bring to the boil.
4. Peel and chop the carrots, sweet potatoes and potatoes and add to the pan. Simmer for 20 minutes.
5. Remove from heat and roughly mash the vegetables.
6. Lay a sheet of filo on a board and cut into two.
7. Place 2 tablespoons of the vegetable mixture on the centre of each piece of filo and fold up corner to corner into a triangle.
8. Pinch the edges together and place on an oiled baking tray.
9. Continue until all the vegetable mixture and filo are used up.
10. Bake in a hot oven, gas mark 4, electric 180C/ 350F, for 30 minutes.

Dip

11. Meanwhile, wash and chop the cucumber into small cubes. Peel and chop the garlic.
12. Add the cucumber, garlic and mint to the soya yoghurt in a bowl. Chill until needed.
13. Serve Yums hot or cold, with a bowl of the dip, salad and potato wedges or other vegetables.

Aubergine and Courgette Fritters with Chilli Dip

This dish is similar to tempura, but I use filo pastry
for the coating so it is much quicker to make.

Serves 2

Dip

　100ml vinegar
　2 tablespoons brown sugar
　2 chopped chillies
　1 tablespoon tomato puree
　2 teaspoons sesame oil
　100ml dry sherry

Fritters

　1 aubergine
　1 courgette
　Sunflower oil to fry
　1 250g pack filo pastry

Dip

1. Warm the vinegar and sugar, stirring until dissolved.
2. Add all the other dip ingredients and simmer for 5 minutes. Cool.

Fritters

3. Slice the aubergine into thin rounds and the courgette into thin strips lengthways.
4. Lay a sheet of filo on a board and cut a piece big enough to wrap a slice of courgette or aubergine two or three times around.
5. Continue until all the vegetable slices have been wrapped.
6. Place a batch of the fritters in a single layer in a frying pan in sunflower oil. Fry for a few minutes each side until browning.
7. Keep the first batch of fritters warm and continue until all the fritters have been cooked.
8. Serve hot with a bowl of the dipping sauce and salad or seasonal vegetables.

(See back cover for photograph)

Catherine Greenall

Aubergine Parmigiana

I don't often use fake cheese, but this is really delicious. It is of course an Italian dish and uses soya-based mozzarella-style cheese.

Serves 2

    1 onion
    6 mushrooms
    5 cloves garlic
    1 400g tin tomatoes
    2 teaspoons basil
    1 teaspoon vegan bouillon
    2 tablespoons tomato puree
    100ml red wine
    1 aubergine
    Olive oil to fry
    200g soya mozzarella

1. Peel, wash and chop the onion, mushrooms and garlic and place in a saucepan.
2. Add the tomatoes, basil, bouillon, tomato puree and red wine and stir.
3. Bring to the boil and simmer for 20 minutes.
4. Cut the stalk from the washed aubergine and slice in half lengthways.
5. Sear the aubergine halves in a frying pan in olive oil for a few minutes on each side.
6. Place the seared aubergine in a small baking dish, cut side up.
7. Add the tomato sauce and top with the sliced mozzarella.
8. Bake for 40 minutes in a hot oven; gas mark 4, electric 180C/ 350F.
9. Serve with salad, vegetables or a little pasta.

Barbequed Aubergine Steaks, Crispy Leeks and Polenta Cakes

The aubergines are braised in a barbeque sauce and served on a bed of crispy fried leeks with polenta cakes.

Serves 2

Barbeque Sauce

- 1 tablespoon brown sugar
- 2 tablespoons soy sauce
- 2 tablespoons dry sherry
- 2 tablespoons balsamic vinegar
- 1 tablespoon lemon juice
- 1 onion
- 2-3 cloves garlic

Aubergine Steaks

- 1 aubergine
- Black pepper
- 1 teaspoon olive oil

Crispy Fried Leeks

- 2 leeks
- 2 teaspoons olive oil
- 1 small piece of ginger root
- 2 cloves garlic

Polenta

- 200g polenta
- 800ml water
- Olive oil to brush over tray

Barbeque Sauce

1. Chop the onion and garlic.
2. Add all the sauce ingredients to a saucepan. Boil then simmer for 5 minutes.

Aubergine Steaks

3. Slice the aubergine lengthways into four thick steaks.
4. Place the aubergine steaks into a baking dish and sprinkle with black pepper.
5. Add the barbeque sauce and marinate in the refrigerator for 3-4 hours.
6. Drizzle with the teaspoon of olive oil.
7. Bake in a hot oven, gas mark 4, electric 180C/ 350F, for 45 minutes.

Crispy Fried Leeks

8. Remove outer leaves and top and tail from the leeks.
9. Cut in half lengthways then across into slices.
10. Place in a colander and wash thoroughly.
11. Heat the 2 teaspoons olive oil in a frying pan, add the chopped leeks.
12. Add the chopped, peeled ginger root and garlic.
13. Fry for 5 minutes.

Polenta Cakes

14. Put the polenta and water into a large pan, mix well and boil then simmer for 5 minutes.
15. Remove from the heat and stand for 10 minutes.
16. Oil a bun tray or Yorkshire pudding tray with olive oil.
17. Pour in the polenta mixture.
18. Bake in a hot oven, gas mark 4, electric 180C/ 350F, for 15 minutes.
    To Serve
19. Place a bed of leeks on each plate and top with the aubergine steaks and barbeque sauce.
20. Serve with the baked polenta cakes.

(See back cover for photograph)

Beancurd, Vegetable and Cashew Nuts in Chilli Sauce with Crispy Fried Aubergine

Make your own delicious Chinese food faster than you can order and collect it from the takeaway!

Serves 2

2 medium carrots
1 courgette
1 green pepper
6 mushrooms
1 bunch spring onions
3 cloves garlic
1 piece of root ginger
1 250g pack beancurd (tofu)
100g cashew nuts
2 teaspoons of olive oil

Crispy Fried Aubergine

Quarter of an aubergine

Chilli Sauce

0.5 cup sherry
2 tablespoons soy sauce
1 teaspoon brown sugar
1 tablespoon wholemeal flour
1 teaspoon chilli powder or 2-3 chopped chillies

1. Finely slice the carrot, courgette, green pepper and mushrooms.
2. Cut the spring onions into 3cm long pieces.
3. Chop the garlic and root ginger
4. Cut the tofu lengthways into slices, then cut each slice into about 3cm strips.
5. Cut the aubergine into thin strips.
6. Mix the sauce ingredients in a cup and stir well.
7. Heat the olive oil in a wok, add tofu and stir fry for 2 minutes. Remove and keep warm.
8. Add the aubergine strips and stir fry until browned and crisp. Remove and keep warm.
9. Add the prepared carrot, courgette, green pepper, mushrooms, spring onions, garlic and root ginger to the wok and stir fry for 3-4 minutes.
10. Add the tofu and cashew nuts to the vegetables in the wok and stir fry for a minute.
11. Add the sauce to the wok and stir well until it bubbles.
12. Serve immediately with boiled rice, topped with the crispy aubergine and soy sauce.

Beer Battered Beetroot

Forget boring pickled beetroot in salads! This is sweet, natural beetroot cooked in a tasty, crispy batter. Delicious served with potato wedges, roasted vegetables and sweet chilli dip.

Serves 2

Beer Batter

4 tablespoons wholemeal flour
0.5 tsp salt
0.5 tsp sugar
1 tsp baking powder
3 tablespoons vegetable oil
120ml beer

Vegetables

2 large cooked beetroot
4 medium potatoes
4 carrots
12 green beans
Sunflower oil
Sweet chilli chutney from a jar to serve

Beer Batter

1. Mix the flour, salt sugar and baking powder in a large bowl or cup.
2. Slowly add the oil and beer, stirring continuously until smooth.
3. Rest batter in refrigerator for 1 hour.

Vegetables

4. Meanwhile, peel, wash and cut the potatoes and carrots in half lengthways then cut each half into two lengthways to form long wedges.
5. Trim and wash the green beans.
6. Place the potato and carrot wedges onto a baking tray and drizzle with sunflower oil.
7. Bake in a hot oven, gas mark 4, electric 180C/ 350F for 45 minutes.
8. After 45 minutes, turn the wedges and add the green beans. Bake at the same temperature for another 15 minutes.
9. Cut the beetroot into thick slices and dip each slice into the beer batter.
10. Place in a single layer in a frying pan containing warmed sunflower oil and fry for a few minutes each side until golden.
11. Keep the first batch of beetroot warm and continue until all the battered beetroot is cooked.
12. Serve the battered beetroot hot, with the vegetable wedges, green beans and sweet chilli chutney.

Beer Battered Tempeh and Asparagus Tips

This is an oriental-inspired dish of tempeh sticks in
a crispy beer batter, served with asparagus tips and
vegetables in a spring onion and ginger sauce.

Serves 2

Beer Batter

    4 tablespoons wholemeal flour
    0.5 tsp salt
    0.5 tsp sugar
    1 tsp baking powder
    3 tablespoons vegetable oil
    120ml beer

Sauce

    100ml dry sherry
    2 tablespoons flour
    2 tablespoons soy sauce
    1 teaspoon ground ginger,
        or small piece of root ginger peeled and chopped
    1 teaspoon Chinese Five Spice

Tempeh and Vegetables

    2 teaspoons olive oil
    6 tempeh sticks
    14 asparagus tips
    6 spring onions
    1 onion
    3 cloves garlic
    75g water chestnuts
    2 portions rice vermicelli

Beer Batter

1. Mix the flour, salt sugar and baking powder in a large bowl or cup.
2. Slowly add the oil and beer, stirring continuously until smooth.
3. Rest batter in refrigerator for 1 hour.

Tempeh and Vegetables

4. Meanwhile, trim and wash the asparagus tips.
5. Trim and wash the spring onions.
6. Peel, wash and chop the onion and garlic.
7. Dip the tempeh sticks into the beer batter until well-coated.
8. Fry tempeh sticks in hot olive oil in a wok for a few minutes each side until golden. Remove and keep warm.
9. Add the asparagus tips to the wok and stir fry for a couple of minutes. Remove and keep warm.
10. Meanwhile, cook the vermicelli according to the manufacturer's instructions.
11. Add the spring onions, onion, garlic and water chestnuts to the wok, with a small amount of additional olive oil, if needed. Stir fry for 2 minutes.
12. Mix all the sauce ingredients in a cup and stir well. Add to the wok and stir for one to two minutes, until the sauce bubbles and thickens.
13. Serve the battered tempeh sticks topped with the asparagus tips, with a portion of vermicelli topped with the vegetables in spring onion and ginger sauce on the side.

(See back cover for photograph)

Bonfire Pie & Red Cabbage

This is based on Lancashire Potato Pie, a warming dish that we always had as children after we returned home cold and sooty from Guy Fawkes Bonfire Night.

Serves 4

Filling

> 1 onion
> 6-8 potatoes
> 2 cups of split red lentils
> 1 teaspoon vegan bouillon
> 0.5 pint water
> Pickled red cabbage to serve

Pastry

> 4 tablespoons flour
> 2 tablespoons vegan margarine
> Approximately 0.3 pint cold water to mix

1. Chop the onion and potatoes into a large saucepan.
2. Add the lentils, water and vegan bouillon.
3. Bring to the boil; then stir and simmer for around 40 minutes until lentils are cooked, checking regularly that the pan does not boil dry. If it becomes too dry, stir in a small amount of water. The filling should be fairly dry in texture at the end of cooking.
4. Meanwhile, place flour and margarine in a mixing bowl.
5. Rub fat into flour until it resembles breadcrumbs.
6. Gradually add water, mixing each time until dough is formed. Knead dough until smooth.
7. Roll out dough on a floured board into a rough circle. Turn half the circle back onto the rolling pin just before use. Make 3 small 45 degree slits in the folded edge, which will be in the centre of the circle when unfolded again. This will allow the pie to 'breathe'.
8. Place cooked filling into a baking dish and top with the pastry circle. Trim off overlapping pastry until about 0.5 inch overlap is left. Double over the overlap into the pastry edges to strengthen the pie crust.
9. Bake for 40 minutes in a hot oven, gas mark 4, electric 180C/ 350F.
10. Serve topped with the red cabbage.

(See back cover for photograph)

Butternut Squash and Spinach Pie

This is a satisfying warming pie, great for serving
with steaming vegetables on cold evenings.

Serves 4

Filling

    1 onion
    2 cloves garlic
    2 teaspoons olive oil
    2 teaspoons curry powder
    1 teaspoon coriander
    ½ teaspoon turmeric
    2 cups of split red lentils
    1 teaspoon vegan bouillon
    0.5 pint water
    1 butternut squash
    100g spinach leaves

Pastry

    10 tablespoons flour
    5 tablespoons vegan margarine
    Approximately 0.5 pint cold water to mix

Filling

1. Chop the onion and garlic into a saucepan and fry in the olive oil for 5 minutes.
2. Add the curry powder, coriander and turmeric and fry for a minute.
3. Add the lentils, water and vegan bouillon.
4. Peel and chop the butternut squash and add to the pan with the washed spinach leaves.
5. Bring to the boil; then stir and simmer for around 40 minutes until lentils are cooked, checking regularly that the pan does not boil dry. If it becomes too dry, stir in a small amount of water. The filling should be fairly dry in texture at the end of cooking.

Pastry

6. Meanwhile, place flour and margarine in a mixing bowl.
7. Rub fat into flour until it resembles breadcrumbs.
8. Gradually add water, mixing each time until dough is formed. Knead dough until smooth.
9. Roll out half the dough on a floured board into a rough circle.
10. Line a pie dish with the pastry. Fold over excess pastry to strengthen the pie edges.
11. Add the cooked butternut squash, spinach and lentils.
12. Roll out the other half of the dough on a floured board into a rough circle.
13. Turn half the circle back onto the rolling pin just before use. Make 3 small 45 degree slits in the folded edge, which will be in the centre of the circle when unfolded again. This will allow the pie to 'breathe'.
14. Place the pastry circle on top of the pie and nip the edges together to seal the pie crust.
15. Bake for 40 minutes in a hot oven, gas mark 4, electric 180C/ 350F.
16. Serve with seasonal vegetables or salad.

Cauliflower and Mushrooms en Croute

In this dish cauliflower is cooked in herb and mushroom sauce; then wrapped in a crispy filo pastry case.

Serves 6

1 cauliflower
6 medium mushrooms
1 red onion
2-3 cloves garlic
2 teaspoons olive oil
2 tablespoons wholemeal flour
½ pint water
1 teaspoon vegan bouillon
1 teaspoon thyme
1 teaspoon basil
1 250g pack filo pastry

1. Cut the cauliflower into florets and wash well.
2. Place in a large pan of water and boil for 5 minutes. Drain and set aside.
3. Peel, wash and chop the mushrooms, red onion and garlic.
4. Fry chopped onion, mushrooms and garlic in olive oil for a few minutes.
5. Add the flour and stir, heating gently until mixed.
6. Gradually add the ½ pint of water, stirring over the heat until sauce begins to bubble and thicken.
7. Add bouillon, thyme and basil and mix well.
8. Line a pie dish with two to three sheets of filo pastry, allowing a lot of overlap over the sides of the dish. Place the pieces of filo at different angles to cover the whole base.
9. Add the blanched cauliflower and cover with the mushroom sauce.
10. Wrap the overlapping pastry across the top of the pie; don't worry about the uneven surface.
11. Brush top with olive oil and bake in a hot oven, gas mark 4, electric 180C/ 350F, for 30-40 minutes until top is browning.
12. Serve hot or cold, with seasonal vegetables or salad.

Catherine Greenall

Crispy Fried Tempeh & Vegetables in Indonesian Satay Sauce

This is based on a dish I first encountered in Holland, which has a large Indonesian community.

Serves 2

6 sticks tempeh
1 onion
3 cloves garlic
2 medium carrots
1 courgette
8 winter cabbage leaves
1 tin or jar of beansprouts
2 teaspoons of olive oil

Satay Sauce

3 tablespoons peanut butter
1 tablespoon soy sauce
1 teaspoon brown sugar
1 tablespoon lemon juice
1 teaspoon chilli powder or 2-3 chopped chillies
1 quarter pint water

To Serve

2 portions vermicelli

1. Chop the onion, garlic, carrots, courgette and cabbage.
2. Mix the sauce ingredients in a saucepan and stir well. Bring to the boil and simmer for 25 minutes.
3. Heat the olive oil in a wok, add tempeh sticks and fry for 2 minutes, turning once. Remove and keep warm.
4. Add the prepared onion, garlic carrots, courgette, beansprouts and cabbage to the wok and stir fry for 3-4 minutes.
5. Meanwhile, cook the vermicelli, according to manufacturer's instructions. This should only take a few minutes.
6. Place a layer of vermicelli on each plate and add the vegetables. Add the crispy tempeh and satay sauce and serve immediately.

(See front cover for photograph)

Devilled Stuffed Portobello Mushrooms

These huge mushrooms look very impressive as a main course.

Serves 2

4 Portobello mushrooms
1 onion
2-3 cloves garlic
2 teaspoons olive oil
4 slices organic wholemeal bread
100g of mixed nuts
1 teaspoon vegan bouillon
1 teaspoon chilli powder or 1 fresh chopped chilli
0.5 pint hot water

1. Remove stalks from washed mushrooms and chop stalks.
2. Fry chopped onion, mushroom stalks and garlic in olive oil for a few minutes until transparent.
3. Meanwhile, make breadcrumbs from the bread in a food processor and transfer to a bowl.
4. Chop mixed nuts in the food processor and add to the bowl.
5. Add the cooked onion mixture.
6. Add stock, made with the hot water and vegan bouillon.
7. Add the chilli and stir well to mix.
8. Place washed mushrooms whole, stalk side up, on an oiled baking tray.
9. Spoon the nut mixture into the mushroom shells.
10. Bake in a hot oven, gas mark 4, electric 180C/ 350F, for 30 minutes.

Dolmades

This is a traditional Greek dish, which can either be served as a snack, or with vegetables or salad as a main course.

Serves 4-6

1 onion
2-3 cloves of garlic
6 mushrooms
100g mixed nuts
2 teaspoons of olive oil
1 cup water
1 teaspoon of vegan bouillon
2 teaspoons of chopped mint leaves
6 tablespoons of long grain rice
0.5 cup sultanas
12 winter cabbage leaves

To finish

1 tablespoon lemon juice
1 cup water
1 teaspoon of vegan bouillon

1. Chop the onion and garlic and slice the mushrooms.
2. Roughly chop the nuts by placing them in a plastic food bag and tapping with a rolling pin.
3. Fry the chopped onion, garlic and mushrooms in the olive oil for a few minutes.
4. Add water, 1 teaspoon vegan bouillon, mint, rice, sultanas and mixed nuts. Simmer for 15 minutes until the rice is cooked and the stock absorbed.
5. Meanwhile, blanch the washed cabbage leaves in boiling water in a large pan for 3 minutes. Drain and cool.
6. Place a cabbage leaf on a large plate or chopping board and place 1 tablespoon of the rice and nut mixture in the middle. Fold up the stalk end, fold in the sides and roll the leaf up into a parcel. Place seam side down in a large baking dish.
7. Continue until all the rice and nut mixture and cabbage leaves are used up, packing them tightly together. Any left-over rice mixture may be frozen when cool.
8. Dissolve the remaining vegan bouillon in the water and pour over the stuffed leaves. Sprinkle with the lemon juice.
9. Bake at gas mark 4, electric 180C/ 350F for 40 minutes.

Eastern Butterbean Casserole

Butterbeans and vegetables infused with eastern
spices and slowly cooked in the oven.

Serves 4

1 onion
2 cloves garlic
2 teaspoons olive oil
1 red pepper
2 sticks celery
2 teaspoons coriander
6 chopped chillies
Juice of 1 lime
0.5 pint water
1 teaspoon vegan bouillon
1 400g tin cooked butterbeans
1 cup (0.4 pints/ 234ml) petit pois
0.5 swede
2lb potatoes

1. Chop the onion and garlic and fry in the olive oil for 2 minutes.
2. Add the chopped red pepper and celery, coriander and chopped chillies
   and stir fry for 2 minutes.
3. Add lime juice, water, vegan bouillon, drained butterbeans and petit
   pois.
4. Bring to the boil.
5. Chop peeled, washed swede and potatoes and place in a large casserole
   dish.
6. Pour the butterbean mixture into the dish and stir. Cover with a lid.
7. Bake for 1.5-2 hours in a hot oven, gas mark 4, electric 180C/ 350F.

Festive Chestnut, Brazil Nut & Brandy Filo Parcels

This makes a great dish for Christmas and other festive occasions.

Serves 6

1 onion
2-3 cloves garlic
4 teaspoons olive oil
8-10 leaves of fresh sage or 2 teaspoons of dried sage
6 slices organic wholemeal bread
250g of Brazil nuts
30 chestnuts
1 teaspoon vegan bouillon
0.5 pint water
30ml brandy
1 250g pack filo pastry

Stuffing

1. Chop the onion and garlic and fry in olive oil for a few minutes until transparent.
2. Add dried or torn-up fresh sage leaves and sweat over low heat for 2 minutes.
3. Wash the chestnuts, slit the skins and boil in a pan of water for 10 minutes.
4. Remove shells whilst still warm.
5. Meanwhile, chop wholemeal bread in a food processor and transfer to a bowl.
6. Chop Brazil nuts in the food processor and add to the bowl.
7. Add the cooked onion and herb mixture and the shelled chestnuts to the bowl.
8. Add 0.5 pint stock, made with the hot water and organic vegan bouillon.
9. Add the brandy.
10. Stir well, mixture should be just moist.

Filo Parcels

11. Lay 2 sheets of filo pastry, one on top of the other, on a chopping board.
12. Cut in half widthways. Place 2 tablespoons stuffing on the centre of each pastry square and fold the edges up into a pocket, pinching the edges together.
13. Place each parcel on an oiled baking tray and brush with olive oil.
14. Continue until all mixture is used; this should make around 12 parcels.
15. Bake in a hot oven, gas mark 4, electric 180C/ 350F, for 30 minutes.
16. Serve with roasted and steamed vegetables.

Lentil Cottage Pie

Serves 4

  1 onion
  2 cloves garlic
  3 carrots
  1 red pepper
  1 cup of split red lentils
  0.5 pint water
  1 teaspoon soy sauce
  1 teaspoon vegan bouillon
  6-8 potatoes
  100ml soya milk
  1 tablespoon vegan margarine

1. Chop the onion, garlic, carrots and pepper into a large saucepan.
2. Add the lentils, water, soy sauce and vegan bouillon.
3. Bring to the boil; then simmer for around 40 minutes until lentils are cooked, checking regularly that the pan does not boil dry. If it becomes too dry, add a small amount of water. The filling should be fairly dry in texture at the end of cooking.
4. Meanwhile, chop potatoes into a pan, add water to cover and boil for 20 minutes.
5. Drain and mash the potatoes, adding soya milk and vegan margarine.
6. Place cooked filling into a baking dish and top with the mashed potatoes.
7. Bake for 40 minutes in a hot oven, gas mark 4, electric 180C/ 350F.

Moroccan Tagine

This dish is named after the pot it is cooked in, which has a lid with a spout. If you do not have one, use an ordinary lidded casserole dish.

Serves 4

1 onion
1 red onion
2 cloves garlic
2 teaspoons olive oil
1 teaspoon cinnamon
2 teaspoons harissa paste
0.5 pint water
1 teaspoon vegan bouillon
1 pinch saffron
1 butternut squash
4 carrots
8 dried figs
1 tablespoon raisins
8 walnut halves

To serve

1 handful flaked almonds
1 handful pistachio nuts

1. Chop the onion and garlic and fry in the olive oil for 2 minutes.
2. Add the cinnamon and harissa and stir fry for 1 minute.
3. Place the fried onions into a tagine pot or casserole dish.
4. Add sliced red onion, water, vegan bouillon, saffron.
5. Add a layer of chopped butternut squash, carrots and dried figs.
6. Cover the dish and place in a hot oven, gas mark 4, electric 180C/ 350F for 20 minutes.
7. Remove from the oven and add the raisins and walnuts.
8. Place in a hot oven, gas mark 4, electric 180C/ 350F for another 15 minutes.
9. Top with the flaked almonds, pistachios and serve with rice or vegetables.

Moussaka

This is based on the traditional Greek dish. The aubergine is fried in olive oil before baking, which gives it a rich flavour.

Serves 4

Vegetable Sauce

1 onion
2-3 cloves of garlic
1 400g tin tomatoes
2 tablespoons tomato puree
1 teaspoon of ground nutmeg
1 teaspoon of vegan organic bouillon
100ml red wine
2 courgettes
4oz mushrooms
Aubergine
Olive oil for frying
2lb potatoes

Bechamel Sauce

1 oz vegan margarine
2 tablespoonfuls wholemeal (or white) flour
0.5 pint soya milk
1 teaspoon vegan bouillon

Vegetable Sauce

1. Add the chopped onion and garlic to a saucepan.
2. Add tomatoes, tomato puree, nutmeg, vegan bouillon and red wine and mix well.
3. Add sliced courgettes and mushrooms. Simmer for 20 minutes.

Aubergine

4. Meanwhile, cut the aubergine into slices. Shallow fry the slices in olive oil in a frying pan in batches, until each side is brown.
5. Put aside on a piece of kitchen towel.

Potatoes

6. Thickly slice potatoes and boil for 5 minutes. Remove from heat and drain.

Bechamel Sauce

7. Melt 1 oz vegan margarine in a saucepan. You could use 1 tablespoon of olive oil instead if preferred.
8. Add two tablespoonfuls of wholemeal (white may be used if preferred) flour. Stir for a few seconds until well mixed.
9. Gradually add soya milk, stirring all the time, whilst gently heating the sauce. The sauce should be fairly thick.
10. Add 1 teaspoon of vegan bouillon.

Assembly

11. Place a layer of potato slices in a large baking dish. Add some of the vegetable sauce on top, then a layer of aubergine slices.
12. Add further layers of potato, vegetable sauce and aubergine. Finish with a layer of potato on the top.
13. Then pour over the béchamel sauce to cover. Sprinkle the top with ground nutmeg.
14. Bake gas mark 4, electric 180C/ 350F for 40 minutes.
15. Serve with seasonal vegetables or salad.

Mung Dal and Mushroom Curry

Mung Dal is made from hulled, split green mung beans and is yellow in colour. Here it is cooked slowly with chillies and spices and served with a cooling mint raita.

Serves 2

1 onion
5 cloves garlic
6 mushrooms
Piece of root ginger
2 teaspoons of olive oil
1 teaspoons coriander or a handful of fresh coriander
2 teaspoons cumin
5 dried or fresh chillies
0.5 pint water
1 teaspoon vegan organic bouillon
1 tablespoon lemon juice
1 cup (234ml) mung dal
Mixed salad leaves
8 cherry tomatoes
200ml soya yoghurt
2 teaspoons chopped mint, or mint in vinegar.
Black pepper

1. Peel and chop the mushrooms, onion, root ginger and garlic.
2. Heat the olive oil in a large pan, add the onions, mushrooms and garlic and stir fry for 2 minutes.
3. Add the root ginger, coriander, cumin and chopped chillies. Fry stirring regularly for a minute
4. Add the water and stir well, bring to the boil.
5. Add the bouillon and mung dal.
6. Mix well and simmer for 1 hour. Check the pan regularly and add a small amount of water if the mixture is getting dry.
7. Meanwhile, make the raita by stirring the mint into the soya yoghurt in a small bowl and top with freshly ground black pepper. Keep in the refrigerator until needed.
8. Wash the salad leaves and tomatoes and arrange in a dish.
9. Add the lemon juice to the cooked mung dal.
10. Serve the mung dal with the boiled rice and the salad and raita as side dishes.

Mushroom & Nut Brandy Parcels with Rainbow Kale

Kale is a highly nutritious curly leafed vegetable, which was used in Roman times. Several colours of kale are available.

Serves 6

1 onion
2-3 cloves garlic
12 mushrooms
2 teaspoons olive oil
6 slices organic wholemeal bread
1 teaspoon parsley
Black pepper
100g of mixed nuts
1 teaspoon vegan bouillon
0.5 pint water
30ml brandy
1 250g pack filo pastry
12-15 leaves of multi-coloured kale
    (or if unavailable, any winter green leaves)

Stuffing

1. Fry chopped onion, mushrooms and garlic in olive oil for a few minutes until transparent.
2. Add parsley and black pepper and sweat over low heat gently for 2 minutes.
3. Meanwhile, make breadcrumbs from the wholemeal bread in a food processor and transfer to a bowl.
4. Chop mixed nuts in the food processor and add to the bowl.
5. Add the cooked onion and herb mixture.
6. Add stock, made with the hot water, vegan bouillon and the brandy.
7. Stir well, mixture should be just moist.

Filo Parcels

8. Lay 2 sheets of filo pastry, one on top of the other, on a chopping board. Cut in half widthways.
9. Place 2 tablespoons stuffing in the middle of each pastry square and fold up pastry edges to form a rough pocket, pinching the edges together. Place each pocket on an oiled baking tray.
10. Continue until all mixture is used; this should make around 12 filo parcels.
11. Bake in a hot oven, gas mark 4, electric 180C/ 350F, for 30 minutes.
12. Meanwhile, wash and steam the kale for around 15 minutes.
13. Serve filo pockets with a small portion of rainbow kale.

(See back cover for photograph)

Mushroom and White Wine Risotto

This is a classic Italian dish made with Arborio
risotto rice and braised in white wine.

Serves 2

1 onion
6 cloves of garlic
2 teaspoons of olive oil
12 mushrooms
10 tablespoons Arborio rice
½ pint water
200ml white wine
1.5 teaspoons vegan organic bouillon
1 teaspoon oregano
1 teaspoon basil
250g jar or tin of petit pois
Sun dried tomatoes from a jar
Freshly ground black pepper
Slivered almonds

1. Peel, wash and chop the onion, mushrooms and garlic.
2. Fry chopped onion, mushrooms and garlic in olive oil for a few minutes.
3. Add the Arborio rice and stir fry for a few seconds.
4. Add water, wine, bouillon, oregano and basil to the pan.
5. Mix well and bring to the boil. Simmer for 25 minutes.
6. Add petit pois and continue to simmer for another 5 minutes.
7. Serve garnished with sun dried tomatoes, slivered almonds and freshly ground black pepper.

Catherine Greenall

Mushroom Quinoa Risotto

This is bursting with proteins and minerals. Quinoa contains all eight essential amino acids and is rich in protein, minerals and Omega 3, 6 and 9.fatty acids

Serves 2

1 onion
2-3 cloves of garlic
2 teaspoons of olive oil
4oz mushrooms
1 400g tin tomatoes
1 teaspoon vegan organic bouillon
1 teaspoon oregano
100ml red wine
12 tablespoons Quinoa
Sun dried tomatoes from a jar
Freshly ground black pepper

1. Chop the onion and garlic.
2. Fry chopped onion and garlic in olive oil for a few minutes.
3. Wash and slice the mushrooms.
4. Add tomatoes, mushrooms, bouillon, oregano and red wine to the pan. Mix well and bring to the boil.
5. Add the Quinoa and simmer for 15 minutes.
6. Serve garnished with sun dried tomatoes and freshly ground black pepper.

Mushrooms and Butter Beans in Red Wine

This is a rich casserole, which can be served with vegetables or rice.

Serves 2

8 mushrooms
1 onion
3 cloves garlic
2 teaspoons of olive oil
1.5 tablespoons flour
100ml water
100ml red wine
0.5 teaspoon thyme
1 teaspoon basil
1 teaspoon oregano
1 teaspoon vegan organic bouillon
1 400g tin of butter beans
Freshly ground black pepper
Fresh basil leaves

1. Chop the mushrooms, onion and garlic.
2. Heat the olive oil in a large saucepan, add the mushrooms, onions and garlic and stir fry for 2 minutes.
3. Add the flour and fry stirring regularly for a minute
4. Gradually add the water and red wine, stirring well over the heat until the sauce is hot and starting to thicken.
5. Add the herbs, bouillon, butter beans and black pepper. Mix well and simmer for 15 minutes.
6. Garnish with the fresh basil leaves and serve with vegetables or rice.

Nut Rolls

These can be served as a main course with salad or vegetables, or as a buffet snack. It is also great for summer picnics and lunchboxes.

Makes 10-12 rolls

Pastry

   10 tablespoons wholemeal flour
   5 tablespoons vegan margarine
   ¼ - ½ pint water to mix

Nut filling

   100g hazelnuts
   100g walnuts
   6 slices organic wholemeal bread
   2 onions
   8 sage leaves
   1 clove garlic
   2 teaspoons olive oil
   1 teaspoon vegan bouillon
   0.5 pint water

Pastry

1. Add flour and vegan margarine to a mixing bowl. Rub fat into flour until it resembles breadcrumbs.
2. Add water in stages, kneading with floured hands, until smooth dough is formed.

Nut Filling

3. Fry chopped onions and garlic in olive oil for a few minutes until transparent.
4. Add sage leaves and sweat over low heat gently for 2 minutes.
5. Meanwhile, make breadcrumbs from the wholemeal bread in a food processor and transfer to a bowl.
6. Chop hazelnuts and walnuts in the food processor and add to the bowl.
7. Add the cooked onion and sage mixture.
8. Add stock, made with the hot water and vegan bouillon.
9. Stir well, mixture should be just moist.

Nut Rolls

10. Roll out half of the pastry into an oblong shape on a floured board.
11. Place half the nut stuffing along the middle of the pastry oblong.
12. Roll up the pastry to form a long roll with the nut filling inside.
13. Cut the roll widthways into 5 or 6 smaller segments and place on an oiled baking tray.
14. Repeat steps 10-13 with the other half of the pastry and nut filling.
15. Bake in a hot oven, gas mark 4, electric 180C/ 350F, for 30 minutes.
16. Serve hot or cold with salad or roasted vegetables.
17. The rolls may also be frozen after step 14. Defrost completely before cooking.

(See back cover for photograph)

Onion & Walnut Tart

This is my version of the French 'Tarte L'Onion'.
Great hot with vegetables as a main dish, or delicious
cold in your picnic or lunchbox. Ooh la la!

Serves 4

Filling

4 onions
2 cloves garlic
4 teaspoons olive oil
0.5 teaspoon brown sugar
1 teaspoon dried basil
0.5 teaspoon oregano
18-20 walnut halves

Pastry

6 tablespoons flour
3 tablespoons vegan margarine
Approximately 0.3 pint cold water

1. Finely slice the onions and garlic.
2. Heat the olive oil in a frying pan and add the onions, garlic, brown sugar, basil and oregano. Fry for 3-5 minutes until the onions are soft.
3. Meanwhile, place flour and margarine in a mixing bowl. Rub fat into flour until it resembles breadcrumbs. Gradually add water, mixing each time. Knead pastry on a floured surface until smooth.
4. Roll out the pastry on a floured board into a rough circle. Place in a pie dish and trim the edges.
5. Place cooked onion mixture into the pastry case and add the walnuts.
6. Bake for 40 minutes in a hot oven, gas mark 4, electric 180C/ 350F.

Pasta with Roasted Vegetables and Mushroom Salsa

This is easy to make, although it takes a little longer
as it involves roasting some vegetables.

Serves 2

½ aubergine
1 courgette
2 teaspoons olive oil to roast
1 red onion
2 cloves garlic
1 400g tin chopped tomatoes
2 chillies
4 mushrooms
2 tablespoons tomato puree
1 teaspoon vegan bouillon
Dried pasta

To Serve

Sun-dried tomatoes from a jar
Freshly ground black pepper

1. Remove the stalk and slice the aubergine across the width into several rounds.
2. Remove the stalk and slice the courgette in half across the width, then lengthways into long slices.
3. Place the aubergine and courgette slices into a baking or roasting dish with the olive oil and roast for 40 minutes in a hot oven, gas mark 4, electric 180C/ 350F
4. Chop the garlic, chillies, mushrooms and onion into a saucepan.
5. Add the tomatoes, tomato puree and bouillon. Bring to the boil and simmer for 20 minutes.
6. Meanwhile, bring about 2 pints of water to the boil in a large saucepan. Add the pasta and boil for 10 minutes, then drain.
7. Mix the pasta with the salsa sauce in the large saucepan.
8. Serve immediately, topped with a stack of the roasted vegetables, sun-dried tomatoes and black pepper.

Penne Pasta with Roasted Vegetables and Pistachios

This is a tasty and colourful Italian dish. Great
if you don't have much time too!

Serves 2

2 courgettes
1 aubergine
2 tomatoes
3 cloves garlic
2 teaspoons of olive oil
Dried penne pasta

Roasted Pistachios

50g pistachio nuts
2 teaspoons olive oil
Sea salt

To Serve

Artichokes from a jar
Fresh basil leaves
Black pepper

1. Cut the courgettes into two and cut each half lengthways into two or three slices.
2. Slice the aubergine across the width into rounds.
3. Cut each tomato into about 6 wedges.
4. Slice the garlic into large pieces.
5. Place 2 teaspoons of olive oil in a baking tray. Add the sliced courgettes, aubergines, tomatoes and garlic, turning the slices in the oil to coat them.
6. Roast in a hot oven gas mark 4, electric 180C/ 350F for around 45 minutes, or until browned.
7. When there is around 10-12 minutes cooking time left, place the other 2 teaspoons of olive oil in a small baking dish. Add the pistachios and sea salt and shake gently to coat the nuts. Roast in a hot oven gas mark 4, electric 180C/ 350F for 10 minutes.
8. Bring about 2 pints of water to the boil in a large saucepan. Add the penne pasta and boil for 10 minutes until the pasta is al dente.
9. Mix the pasta with the roasted vegetables in the baking dish.
10. Serve immediately; topped with the roasted pistachios, artichokes, fresh basil and black pepper.

Penne with Tomato & Garlic Sauce

This is really easy and very garlicky, so make
sure your friends have some too!

Serves 2

6 cloves garlic
1 onion
2 teaspoons of olive oil
1 400g tin chopped tomatoes
2 tablespoons tomato puree
1 teaspoon oregano
1 teaspoon vegan bouillon
Dried penne pasta

To Serve

Sun-dried tomatoes from a jar
Sliced almonds
Black pepper

1. Chop the garlic and onion into a saucepan with the olive oil. Fry gently for 2 minutes.
2. Add the tomatoes, tomato puree, oregano and bouillon. Bring to the boil and simmer for 15 minutes.
3. Meanwhile, bring about 2 pints of hot water from the kettle back to the boil in a large saucepan. Add the pasta and boil for 10 minutes.
4. Drain the pasta and toss in the tomato and garlic sauce.
5. Serve immediately, topped with the sliced almonds, sun-dried tomatoes and black pepper.

Porcini Mushroom Risotto

Porcini is the Italian name for this gourmet mushroom, which is also known as cep in France or boletus. Fresh porcini can be expensive, but you can use dried as in this recipe.

Serves 2

20g dried porcini mushrooms
100ml red wine
1 400g tin chopped tomatoes
1 onion
2 cloves of garlic
1 teaspoon vegan organic bouillon
2 tablespoons tomato puree
10 tablespoons Arborio rice

To serve

Fresh basil leaves
Freshly ground black pepper
Olives
Slivered almonds

1. Soak the porcini mushrooms, just covered with hot water from the kettle, in a small bowl for 4 hours.
2. Peel, wash and chop the onion and garlic into a large saucepan.
3. Add the soaked mushrooms with the steeping liquid.
4. Add the red wine, tomatoes, bouillon, tomato puree and Arborio rice.
5. Mix well and bring to the boil. Simmer for 30 minutes. Add a little more water if the mixture starts to dry out.
6. Serve garnished with olives, basil leaves, slivered almonds and freshly ground black pepper.

Puy Lentil and Mushroom Curry

Mushrooms and vegetables are gently simmered with puy
lentils in an aromatic sauce with Indian spices.

Serves 2

8 mushrooms
1 onion
5 cloves garlic
2 teaspoons of olive oil
1 teaspoons curry powder
1 teaspoons coriander or a handful of fresh coriander
2 teaspoons cumin
0.5 teaspoon turmeric
0.5 pint water
1 teaspoon vegan organic bouillon
1 tablespoon lemon juice
1 cup puy lentils
2 potatoes
1 carrot
¼ cabbage
Chappatis or tortillas
Rice

1. Chop the mushrooms, onion and garlic.
2. Peel and chop potatoes and carrots into small pieces
3. Wash the cabbage and cut into shreds.
4. Heat the olive oil in a large pan, add the onions, mushrooms and garlic and stir fry for 2 minutes.
5. Add the curry powder, coriander, cumin and turmeric. Fry stirring regularly for a minute
6. Add the water and stir well, bring to the boil.
7. Add the bouillon, lemon juice, potatoes, carrots, cabbage and puy lentils.
8. Mix well and simmer for 50 minutes.
9. Fold the chappatis or tortillas into halves then quarters and wrap in foil. Warm in a hot oven, gas mark 4, electric 180C/ 350F, for 5 minutes.
10. Serve curry with the warmed chappatis and boiled rice.

Refried Bean Tortillas

I like to make this Mexican dish on Pancake
Day as a savoury main course.

Serves 2

1 red onion
5 cloves garlic
2 teaspoons olive oil
1 teaspoon ground coriander
4 chopped chillies
1 400g tin of kidney beans, drained
2 tablespoons water
½ teaspoon vegan bouillon
2 flour tortillas
6 tablespoons soya yoghurt
Salad leaves

1. Peel and chop the red onion and garlic and fry in the olive oil for 2 minutes.
2. Add the coriander, beans and chopped chillies and stir fry for 2 minutes.
3. Add water and vegan bouillon and simmer for 5 minutes.
4. Meanwhile, wrap the tortillas in foil and heat for 5 minutes in a hot oven, gas mark 4, electric 180C/ 350F.
5. Lay a tortilla flat on each large plate.
6. Place 3-4 tablespoons of the refried beans along the middle of each tortilla and roll up.
7. Top with the soya yoghurt and serve immediately with salad.

Rich Vegetable Chilli

If you like it hot; try this!

Serves 2

1 onion
3 cloves garlic
6 mushrooms
1 courgette
2 teaspoons of olive oil
1 teaspoon coriander
1 400g tin of chopped tomatoes
1 400g tin of kidney beans, drained
1 400g tin black beans
1 400g tin baked beans
4-6 chillies
1 teaspoon vegan organic bouillon
1 cup soya mince (or 100g finely chopped walnuts)
100 ml red wine
1 avocado

1. Chop the mushrooms, courgette, onion and garlic.
2. Chop the chillies separately.
3. If using walnuts, chop finely in a food processor.
4. Heat the olive oil in a large saucepan, add the mushrooms, courgette, onion and garlic and fry for 2 minutes.
5. Add coriander and fry for a minute.
6. Add the tomatoes, kidney beans, baked beans and black beans, chillies, bouillon, soya mince (or walnuts) and red wine. Mix well and simmer for 15 minutes.
7. Meanwhile peel, stone and chop the avocado. Place in a bowl with a sprinkling of lemon juice.
8. Serve with boiled rice and garnish with the chopped avocado.

Roasted Vegetable Pizza

Who said pizza has to contain cheese? This is not only delicious, it's much healthier! It also makes your kitchen smell divine.

Serves 4

Pizza Base

   10 tablespoons flour
   2 tablespoons olive oil
   1 pinch of sea salt
   1 sachet of quick action yeast (or other dried yeast)
   0.5 pint warm water
       (mix hot water from the kettle with cold water from the tap)

Topping Base

   1 400g tin chopped tomatoes
   1 onion
   2 cloves garlic
   1 teaspoon oregano
   2 tablespoons tomato puree

Roasted vegetables

   1 courgette
   1 aubergine
   2 teaspoons olive oil for roasting

To Finish

   Sliced almonds
   6 sun dried tomatoes
   10 olives
   1 teaspoon olive oil
   Black pepper from a pepper mill

Catherine Greenall

Pizza Base

1. Place flour and salt in a warmed mixing bowl.
2. Add olive oil and rub in with fingertips until absorbed.
3. Add the yeast and mix, then add the warm water gradually, mixing with floured hands each time.
4. Knead with floured hands on a floured surface for 5 minutes until bread dough is smooth and elastic.
5. Place in a floured bowl, covered with a clean cloth, in a warm place and leave for around 1 hour until doubled in size.
6. Knead again for 5 minutes on a floured surface with floured hands. Oil a pizza tray and work the dough into the tray, manipulating into a large circle with floured hands, or use a rolling pin.
7. Leave covered with a clean cloth in the pizza tray in a warm place for one hour.

Roasted vegetables

8. Slice the courgette and aubergine and place in a roasting tray with the olive oil. Roast in a hot oven gas mark 4, electric 180C/ 350F for 30 minutes.

Topping Base

9. Chop the onion and garlic into a saucepan. Add the tinned tomatoes, tomato puree and oregano and simmer for 20 minutes.

To assemble

10. Spread the tomato base over the pizza dough.
11. Arrange the roasted vegetables, sliced almonds, sun dried tomatoes and olives on the top.
12. Drizzle with the olive oil and add freshly ground black pepper.
13. Bake for around 30 minutes in a hot oven gas mark 4, electric 180C/ 350F.

(See back cover for photograph)

Roasted Vegetable Polenta Tart

Polenta is made from maize and is an ancient Italian food that was eaten by Roman soldiers. Low in fat, it is a good source of fibre, carbohydrate, protein and iron.

Serves 4-6

Pastry

4 tablespoons wholemeal flour
2 tablespoons vegan margarine
Cold water to mix (around $^1/3$ - ½ pint)

Filling

60g polenta
½ pint soya milk
1 teaspoon vegan bouillon
1 aubergine
2 courgettes
Olive oil for roasting
1 onion
2 cloves garlic
2 teaspoons olive oil
Chopped chives

1. Place the flour and margarine in a mixing bowl and rub fat into flour until it resembles breadcrumbs.
2. Add water slowly, mixing in with floured hands and knead until an elastic dough forms.
3. Roll out the pastry on a floured board, place in a greased baking tin and bake for 15 minutes in a hot oven; gas mark 4, electric 180C/ 350F.
4. Slice the aubergine into thick rounds and the courgette into thick strips lengthways. Place in a baking tray with olive oil to coat and roast for 30 minutes in a hot oven; gas mark 4, electric 180C/ 350F.
5. Meanwhile, add the polenta, bouillon and soya milk to a saucepan and bring to the boil. Simmer for 5 minutes, then leave to stand for 10 minutes.
6. Peel and chop the onion and garlic and fry in the olive oil for 2 minutes.
7. Remove the pastry case from the oven and top with the onion and garlic.
8. Pour the polenta into the pastry case whilst still warm.
9. Arrange the roasted aubergine and courgette slices on top of the tart and add the chopped chives. (You could delay the rest of the cooking at this stage if desired.)
10. Drizzle with a tablespoon of olive oil and bake for 40 minutes in a hot oven; gas mark 4, electric 180C/ 350F.
11. Serve hot or cold with salad or seasonal vegetables.

(See back cover for photograph)

Sag Aloo Channa Sabzi

This is an Indian curry with spinach, chick peas and vegetables.

Serves 2

6 mushrooms
2 carrots
1 courgette
1 onion
3 cloves garlic
1 head of broccoli
2 potatoes
100g spinach leaves
2 teaspoons of olive oil
2 teaspoons curry powder
2 teaspoons coriander or a handful of fresh coriander
1 teaspoon cumin
0.5 teaspoon turmeric
0.5 pint water
1 400g can chick peas
1 teaspoon vegan organic bouillon
50g slice creamed coconut
Fresh coriander to garnish

1. Slice the mushrooms, carrots, courgette, onion and garlic.
2. Break washed broccoli into small florets.
3. Chop potatoes into small pieces
4. Wash the spinach
5. Heat the olive oil in a large pan, add the onions and garlic and stir fry for 2 minutes.
6. Add the curry powder, coriander, cumin and turmeric. Fry stirring regularly for a minute
7. Add the water and stir well, bring to the boil.
8. Add the bouillon, coconut, mushrooms, carrots, courgette, broccoli, potatoes, spinach and chick peas.
9. Mix well and simmer for 20 minutes.
10. Garnish with fresh coriander and serve with boiled or steamed rice.

Spaghetti Pesto Duo Colore

This is a two-colour pesto, made from green basil leaves and red tomatoes. I like to make my own pesto; it is so much nicer. But beware it is very garlicky, so only eat this if you are staying in!

Serves 2

2 tablespoons olive oil
3 cloves garlic
Pinch of sea salt
50g pine nuts
Large handful of washed, fresh basil leaves
4-6 sun dried tomatoes
Dried spaghetti

To Serve

Sun-dried tomatoes from a jar
Freshly ground black pepper

1. Bring about 2 pints of water to the boil in a large saucepan. Add the spaghetti and boil for 10 minutes.
2. Meanwhile, place the garlic, olive oil, sea salt, pine nuts, basil leaves and 4-6 sun dried tomatoes in a food processor. Whiz until mixed to a paste.
3. Serve the spaghetti immediately, topped with the pesto sauce, sun-dried tomatoes and black pepper.

Spinach and Spring Onion Tart

This tart is great hot or cold, with vegetables or salad as a main course. It is also good in picnics and lunch boxes.

Serves 4-6

Pastry

> 4 tablespoons wholemeal flour
> 2 tablespoons vegan margarine
> Cold water to mix (around $1/3$ - ½ pint)

Filling

> 6 spring onions
> 200g spinach leaves
> 180g polenta
> 500ml water
> 2 teaspoon vegan bouillon
> Freshly ground black pepper
> 2 teaspoons olive oil

1. Place the flour and margarine in a mixing bowl and rub fat into flour until it resembles breadcrumbs.
2. Add water slowly, mixing in with floured hands and knead until an elastic dough forms.
3. Roll out the pastry on a floured board and line a greased pie dish with the pastry.
4. Top and tail the spring onions, wash and chop. Add to the pastry case.
5. Wilt the washed spinach leaves in a saucepan, just with the water which clings to them, for 5 minutes on low heat. Add to the pastry case.
6. Add the polenta, bouillon and water to a saucepan and bring to the boil. Simmer for 5 minutes, then leave to stand for 10 minutes.
7. Pour the polenta into the pastry case whilst still warm.
8. Drizzle top with the olive oil, add black pepper and bake for 40 minutes in a hot oven; gas mark 4, electric 180C/ 350F.
9. Serve hot or cold with salad or seasonal vegetables.

Catherine Greenall

Sweet Potato, Lentil and Spinach Nut Crumble

This makes an excellent Sunday lunch,
packed with protein and vitamins.

Serves 4

Filling

1 onion
2-3 cloves of garlic
2 teaspoons of olive oil
2 teaspoon of curry powder
1 half teaspoon of turmeric
0.5 pint water
1 teaspoon organic vegan bouillon
2 small (or 1 large) chopped sweet potatoes
100g washed spinach leaves
1 cup of split red lentils

Nut Crumble

6 tablespoons wholemeal organic flour
3 tablespoons non-dairy spread
100g walnuts

Filling

1. Fry the chopped onion and garlic in the olive oil for a few minutes in a large pan.
2. Add curry powder and turmeric and fry for a few seconds, stirring.
3. Add water, vegan bouillon (or other vegetable stock), the sweet potatoes, spinach and lentils.
4. Bring to the boil; then simmer for around 40 minutes until lentils are cooked, checking regularly that the pan does not boil dry. The mixture should be fairly dry at the end, but if it becomes too dry whilst cooking, add a small amount of water from the kettle.

Walnut Crumble

5. Add flour and non-dairy spread to a large mixing bowl.
6. Rub fat into flour until it resembles breadcrumbs.
7. Roughly crumble the walnuts into the crumble mix.

Assembly

8. Place the filling mixture in a large baking dish and top with the crumble so that the filling is completely covered.
9. Bake in a hot oven gas mark 4, electric 180C/ 350F for 40 minutes.
10. Serve with steamed and roasted seasonal vegetables.

Catherine Greenall

Ten-Minute Spaghetti Supper

So you think you have no time to cook tonight? This literally only takes ten minutes, from the time the kettle boils – and it tastes great!

Serves 2

Dried spaghetti
3 cloves garlic
2 dried or fresh chillies
2 teaspoons of olive oil

Roasted Pistachios

50g pistachio nuts
2 teaspoons olive oil
Sea salt

To Serve

Artichokes and olives from a jar
Fresh basil leaves
Black pepper

1. Bring about 2 pints of hot water from the kettle back to the boil in a large saucepan. Add the spaghetti and boil for 10 minutes.
2. Make the roasted pistachios by placing 2 teaspoons of olive oil in a small baking dish. Add the pistachios and sea salt and shake gently to coat the nuts. Roast in a hot oven, gas mark 4, electric 180C/ 350F for 10 minutes.
3. Meanwhile, chop the garlic and chillies into a small saucepan with the other 2 teaspoons of olive oil. Fry gently for 5 minutes.
4. Drain the spaghetti and toss in the garlic, oil and chilli mixture.
5. Serve immediately, topped with the roasted pistachios, olives, artichokes, fresh basil and black pepper.

Thai Beancurd and Vegetable Green Curry

This is a pretty hot Thai dish. You could always
reduce the chillies if you like a milder dish.

Serves 2

1 250g pack beancurd (tofu)
1 red pepper
6 mushrooms
1 head of broccoli
1 bunch spring onions
3 cloves garlic
1 piece of root ginger
2 teaspoons of olive oil
2 teaspoons chilli powder or 6 chopped fresh chillies
2 teaspoons coriander or a handful of fresh coriander
1 teaspoon galangal powder
0.5 teaspoon turmeric
1 400ml tin of coconut milk
Juice of 1 lime
2 teaspoons Thai Holy Basil
1 teaspoon chopped lemongrass
1 teaspoon vegan organic bouillon

1. Cut the tofu lengthways into slices, then cut each slice into about 3cm strips.
2. Finely slice the red pepper and mushrooms.
3. Cut the washed broccoli into small florets.
4. Cut the spring onions into 3cm long pieces.
5. Chop the peeled garlic and root ginger
6. Heat the olive oil in a large pan, add the prepared spring onions and garlic and stir fry for 2 minutes.
7. Add the chilli powder or fresh chillies, coriander, galangal powder and turmeric. Fry stirring regularly for a minute
8. Add the coconut milk and stir well, bring to the boil.
9. Add the lime juice, Thai Holy Basil, lemongrass, bouillon, red pepper, mushrooms, broccoli, tofu, and root ginger.
10. Mix well and simmer for 10 minutes.
11. Serve with boiled or steamed fragrant rice.

Three Bean Casserole

Mixed beans and vegetables are cooked gently
in a rich herb and tomato sauce.

Serves 4

1 onion
4 cloves garlic
2 sticks celery
2 carrots
400g tin red kidney beans
400g tin chick peas
1 cup (234mls) yellow split peas
400g tin tomatoes
1 teaspoon basil
1 teaspoon oregano
1 teaspoon cumin
2 tablespoons tomato puree
0.5 pint water
1 teaspoon vegan bouillon

1. Peel and chop the onion, garlic, celery and carrots.
2. Place chopped vegetables in a large saucepan.
3. Add all the other ingredients, bring to the boil then simmer for 2 hours.
4. Serve either with a chunk of bread as a snack, or with vegetables as a main course.

Chapter 4:
'Sorry, You Can't Have Any of These'
Delicious Desserts

Most restaurants' dessert menus consist of creamy gateaux, sticky toffee puddings, roulades and ice cream sundaes. Hey, you might strike lucky - they may do a fresh fruit salad! But if you get bored with that, try some of these.

Baked Polenta Custard Tart

I used to love custard pie as a child. This has a firmer texture but the flavours are similar.

Serves 4-6

Pastry

> 6 tablespoons organic white (or wholemeal) flour
> 3 tablespoons vegan margarine
> 0.5 cup water

Filling

> 60g polenta
> 1 tablespoon vanilla extract
> 2 tablespoons brown sugar
> ½ pint soya milk
> Pinch ground nutmeg

1. Make the pastry by rubbing the fat into the flour in a mixing bowl. When the mixture resembles breadcrumbs, add a little of the water and continue mixing with floured hands. Continue to add water and knead until the pastry is elastic and smooth. Roll out the pastry on a floured board using a rolling pin.
2. Line a greased pie dish with the pastry. Bake blind for 15 minutes in a hot oven, gas mark 4, electric 180C/ 350F. This means adding a circle of foil or greaseproof paper onto the top of the pastry and then dried peas or beans to weigh down the pastry.
3. Meanwhile, heat the soya milk until it just boils.
4. Add the polenta, vanilla extract and brown sugar. Mix well and simmer gently for 5 minutes. Remove from heat and stand for 10 minutes.
5. Remove pastry from oven and take out the foil and beans or peas.
6. Pour in the polenta mixture and top with the ground nutmeg.
7. Bake for a further 35 minutes in a hot oven, gas mark 4, electric 180C/ 350F.
8. Cut into slices and serve hot or cold.

(See back cover for photograph)

Blackberry Sorbet

This is a great companion to the Normandy Apple Tart.

Makes enough to fill a 400ml tub

2 tablespoons of water
2 tablespoons of brown sugar
2 tablespoons lemon juice
300ml red wine
80ml Cassis
400g blackberries

1. Heat the water, sugar and lemon juice in a saucepan, stirring until the sugar is dissolved.
2. Add the red wine and cassis and cool.
3. Puree the blackberries in a food processor and strain through a sieve.
4. Return the sieved blackberries with the red wine mixture to the food processor and blend, then place in a plastic tub with a lid.
5. Place in the freezer for 1 hour, then remove and beat well or blend again.
6. Repeat step 5. This stops large crystals from forming and produces a smooth sorbet.
7. Remove sorbet from freezer 30 minutes before serving.

(See front cover for photograph)

Blueberry and Raspberry Cheesecake

This dessert is delicious served chilled.

Serves 4-6

Fruit Topping

40 raspberries – fresh or frozen
150g blueberries
1.5 tablespoons brown sugar
3 tablespoons red wine

Biscuit Base

150g plain vegan biscuits (lemon or ginger ones work well)
50g creamed coconut
1 tablespoon vegetable oil

Cream Topping

250g plain tofu
1 tablespoon brown sugar
50g creamed coconut
1 tablespoon vanilla extract

Fruit Topping

1. Reserve 10 raspberries for decoration. Place the remaining raspberries in a saucepan with the blueberries.
2. Add the brown sugar and red wine.
3. Bring to the boil and then simmer for 15minutes. The mixture should be quite jammy. Allow the fruit to cool.

Base

4. Place the biscuits in a large plastic food bag and crush using a rolling pin.
5. Melt the creamed coconut with the oil in a small saucepan.
6. Add the biscuit crumbs and mix well.
7. Transfer to a loose base baking tin and press down until compact.

Cream Topping

8. Melt the creamed coconut in a small saucepan.
9. Place the tofu, sugar, melted creamed coconut and vanilla extract into a food processor and blitz until smooth.

Assembly

10. Place the cream topping on top of the biscuit base.
11. Top with the cooled raspberries and blueberries.
12. Decorate with the reserved raspberries.
13. Chill for 3-4 hours before serving.

(See back cover for photograph)

Chocolate Cakes with Brandied Summer Fruits

Makes 12

Chocolate Cakes

> 6 squares organic dark chocolate
> 5oz vegan margarine
> 5oz sugar
> 1 tablespoon cocoa powder
> 5oz organic white flour
> 1 teaspoon baking powder
> Soya milk

Brandied Summer Fruits

> 200g summer fruits (fresh or frozen)
> 100ml brandy

Brandied Summer Fruits

1. Place the summer fruits in a large bowl and mix in the brandy.
2. Marinate in a refrigerator for 2-4 hours.

Chocolate Cakes

1. Oil a 12-portion non-stick bun tray.
2. Melt the chocolate squares in a bowl over a small pan of boiling water. Do not let the water come into contact with the chocolate.
3. In a mixing bowl, cream together the margarine and sugar using a fork.
4. Add the melted chocolate and mix well.
5. Add the cocoa powder and flour and mix well.
6. Moisten with a little soya milk and mix until creamy.
7. Spoon the mixture into the bun tray and bake for around 15 minutes at 150C/300F/ gas mark 3, until firm to the touch.
8. Cool; then place in an airtight tin until use.

To Serve

1. Place a chocolate cake on each plate.
2. Top each cake with the brandied summer fruits and serve with vegan sorbet or ice-cream, if liked.

Catherine Greenall

Cinnamon Bananas and Blueberries

Blueberries are one of the richest sources of antioxidants, which help to reduce the effects of aging and lower the risk of cancer.

Serves 2

2 bananas
2 large handfuls of blueberries – fresh or frozen
4 tablespoons water
1 tablespoon brown sugar
1 teaspoon vanilla extract
2 teaspoons sesame oil
Ground cinnamon
Soya yoghurt

1. Peel the bananas and cut each in half, then cut each half lengthways
2. Place cut side up in a baking dish.
3. Add the water, sugar, vanilla and sesame oil. Sprinkle the top with cinnamon.
4. Bake in a hot oven, gas mark 4, electric 180C/ 350F for 20 minutes.
5. Arrange bananas in a dish whilst still warm and add the blueberries.
6. Serve warm or cold topped with soya yoghurt.

Mango and Lime Sorbet

Sorbet is a great alternative to ice cream, as it has very few calories and if you make your own, no additives!

Makes enough to fill a 400ml tub

½ pint (300ml) water
80ml Schnapps (or any clear spirit)
2 tablespoons of brown sugar
4 tablespoons lime juice
1 teaspoon ground ginger
1 mango

1. Heat the water, schnapps, sugar, lime juice and ginger in a saucepan, stirring until the sugar is dissolved.
2. Peel and chop the mango and add to the saucepan. Simmer for 10 minutes.
3. Cool the mixture completely. Mix in a blender or food processor and place in a plastic tub.
4. Place in the freezer for 1 hour, then remove and beat well or blend again.
5. Repeat step 4. This stops large crystals from forming and produces a smooth sorbet.
6. Remove sorbet from freezer 30 minutes before serving. Serve as it is or topped with berries.

Normandy Apple Tart

This is great way of using the apple harvest, with a French twist – only for the adults! Calvados brandy is produced from apples in the Normandy region of France.

Serves 4

Topping

6 baking apples
50g sultanas
25g dried blueberries
50ml Calvados
1-2 tablespoon of brown sugar
Cinnamon to dust
2 tablespoons of icing sugar to decorate

Pastry

6 tablespoons organic white (or wholemeal) flour
3 tablespoons vegan margarine
0.5 cup water

1. Soak the sultanas and blueberries overnight in the Calvados, in a bowl kept in the refrigerator. You could substitute Calvados with fruit juice.
2. Make the pastry by rubbing the fat into the flour in a mixing bowl. When the mixture resembles breadcrumbs, add a little of the water and continue mixing with floured hands. Continue to add water and knead until the pastry is elastic and smooth. Roll out the pastry on a floured board using a rolling pin. Line a greased pie dish with the pastry.
3. Core, peel and slice the apples. Place sliced apples on top of the pastry base until completely covered. Top with the soaked fruits and sprinkle with the brown sugar and cinnamon.
4. Bake for 35 minutes in a hot oven, gas mark 4, electric 180C/ 350F.
5. Place icing sugar in a sieve or perforated shaker.
6. Cut the tart into slices and decorate with a dusting of icing sugar.
7. Serve hot or cold with blackberry sorbet.

(See front cover for photograph)

Poached Pears in Red Wine

This is an easy but impressive-looking dessert.

Serves 4

4 pears
1 teaspoon of cinnamon
1 tablespoon of brown sugar
500 ml of red wine
10 raspberries
2 tablespoons of icing sugar

1. Core and peel the pears, leave whole.
2. Place pears upright in a saucepan just large enough to hold them.
3. Add the cinnamon, brown sugar and red wine and stir well.
4. Bring to the boil and simmer for 15-20 minutes, until pears are soft.
5. Remove the pears and place in a covered dish to cool.
6. Simmer the remaining liquid until it becomes syrupy and thick. You will need to watch the pan carefully whilst the liquid is reduced down, as it could solidify or burn. When it is just thick enough to coat the back of a spoon, pour into a small jug or bowl and cool.
7. Arrange the pears on a plate.
8. Place icing sugar in a sieve or perforated shaker.
9. Decorate with the red wine syrup, raspberries and a dusting of icing sugar.

Pecan and Blueberry Granola

You can serve this with soya milk for breakfast, or
sprinkled on sorbet or fresh fruit for added crunch.

500g porridge oats
4 tablespoons of brown sugar
120ml sunflower oil
200g pecans
100g dried blueberries

1. Mix the oats, sugar and sunflower oil in a large baking dish.
2. Bake in a hot oven, gas mark 4, electric 180C/ 350F for 15 minutes.
3. Remove from oven and add the pecans, mix well.
4. Return to the oven and bake for a further 15 minutes.
5. Remove from oven and cool. Add the blueberries and mix well.
6. The granola can be stored in a plastic tub and should keep for a few
    weeks.
7. Serve with soya milk or as a topping for desserts.

Pineapple and Raspberry Stack

This is a tropical-influenced dessert that looks
impressive, but is really easy to make.

Serves 2

8 slices of fresh pineapple
100ml red or white rum
Raspberries – fresh or frozen
Soya yoghurt to serve
Icing sugar to dust

1. Soak the sliced pineapple in the rum for about four hours.
2. Pile the pineapple slices into stacks and drizzle with the rum used for the marinade.
3. Decorate with the raspberries.
4. Sprinkle with icing sugar and serve with soya yoghurt.

Quick Raspberry Pancakes

I often make this as a dessert on Pancake Tuesday – but
you don't have to wait until then to enjoy it!

Serves 2

2 ready-made flour tortillas
Raspberries – fresh or frozen
Soya yoghurt
Icing sugar to dust

1. Wrap the tortillas in foil and warm in a hot oven, gas mark 4, electric 180C/ 350F for 5 minutes.
2. Remove foil and fill each tortilla with raspberries whilst still warm and roll up.
3. Sprinkle with icing sugar and serve warm topped with soya yoghurt.

Catherine Greenall

Raspberry and Blueberry Delight

You could use any seasonal berries, soaked in your favourite liqueur here.

Serves 2

    Raspberries – fresh or frozen
    Blueberries – fresh or frozen
    100ml blackcurrant liqueur or cassis
    1-2 vegan biscuits
    2 scoops mango and lime sorbet

1. Place layers of raspberries, then blueberries into 2 sundae glasses.
2. Drizzle over the blackcurrant liqueur or cassis and marinate for 2 hours in a refrigerator.
3. Add a scoop of mango and lime sorbet to each glass.
4. Place the vegan biscuits in a plastic food bag and crush with a rolling pin.
5. Top each glass with the crushed biscuit and serve.

Rhubarb and Apple Cranachan

Cranachan is a traditional Scottish dessert. I have used soya yoghurt in place of whipped cream and brown sugar in place of honey. It is usually made with raspberries, but any seasonal soft fruit can be used.

Serves 2

Fruit layer

- 1 stick of rhubarb
- 2 eating apples
- 5 tablespoons water
- 1 tablespoon vanilla extract
- 1 tablespoon brown sugar

Toasted Oatmeal

- 8 tablespoons oats
- 1 tablespoon brown sugar
- 2 tablespoons sunflower oil
- 0.5 teaspoon cinnamon

Topping

- 200ml soya yoghurt
- 2 tablespoons whisky
- 1 tablespoon brown sugar

Catherine Greenall

Fruit layer

1. Peel and chop the rhubarb and apples into a saucepan.
2. Add water, vanilla extract and brown sugar and simmer for 15 minutes.

Toasted Oats

3. Mix the oats, sugar, sunflower oil and cinnamon in a baking tray.
4. Bake for 40 minutes in a hot oven, gas mark 4, electric 180C/ 350F.

Topping

5. Mix the soya yoghurt and whisky in a bowl.
6. Add brown sugar to taste.

To Serve

7. Place a layer of the fruit in a bowl or sundae glass.
8. Top with the toasted oats and serve with the whisky yoghurt.

Rhubarb, Ginger and Plum Trifle

English trifle originated in the 1700s as a way of using up stale cake, which is soaked in sherry and layered with fruit, custard and whipped cream.

Serves 4

2 sticks of rhubarb
4 plums
50ml brandy
50ml water
1 tablespoon brown sugar
1 teaspoon cinnamon
100ml sherry
8 vegan ginger biscuits
200ml soya yoghurt

1. Peel and chop the rhubarb into a saucepan with the plums.
2. Add the water, brandy, cinnamon and brown sugar and simmer for 15 minutes. Cool.
3. Take four sundae dishes and place a plum in the base of each.
4. Pour the sherry into a shallow bowl or plate.
5. Dip four biscuits one by one into the sherry and quickly break one into each sundae dish.
6. Add a tablespoon of soya yoghurt into each dish.
7. Divide the rhubarb mixture between the sundae dishes.
8. Dip the remaining four biscuits one by one into the sherry and then add to each a sundae dish.
9. Top with soya yoghurt, chill and serve.

Catherine Greenall

Tipsy Blueberry Fool

Fruit fool is an English dish that dates from the sixteenth century. It consists of sweetened fruit, traditionally gooseberries, folded into whipped cream.

Serves 2

200g blueberries – fresh or frozen
200ml port
200ml soya yoghurt
4 squares organic dark chocolate

1. Place the dark chocolate in the refrigerator until required.
2. Wash the blueberries and place into 2 sundae glasses.
3. Drizzle the port over the berries.
4. Chill for four hours.
5. Top each glass with soya yoghurt and partially mix with the blueberries.
6. Grate the dark chocolate.
7. Add the grated dark chocolate topping and serve.

(See back cover for photograph)

Chapter 5: 'What Do You Eat?'

This is usually the next thing that people say when you have just given them the list of things that are off your menu. Actually, as you probably know (unless you are reading this in a panic because your significant other, family member or friend has suddenly gone vegan) there are loads of things you can eat, some of which even normal people eat!

Vegans do not eat any animal or fish flesh or products obtained from them. This includes dairy products, eggs and honey. In addition, they do not use animal products for clothing (leather, silk, wool, fur) or cosmetics.

You do need to be aware of nutritional needs and ensure you have a balanced diet.

Nutrition

It is perfectly possible to maintain a healthy diet whilst following a vegan lifestyle. In order to achieve this, you need to include protein, fruit, vegetables, legumes, seeds, nuts and wholefoods. This includes young and older adults and children. As some groups have specific nutritional requirements, you may wish to check for additional information on the web-sites listed in Chapter 6.

Antioxidants

Studies have indicated that antioxidants may protect cells from the damage caused by molecules known as free radicals. Free radical damage may lead to cancer, heart and other aging-related illnesses. Sources of antioxidants include fruits, vegetables, whole grains and nuts. Examples are carrots, tomatoes, green leafy vegetables, Brazil nuts and citrus fruits.

Calcium

Calcium helps to form strong bones. Sources include Brazil nuts, green leafy vegetables and fortified tofu and soya milk.

Fat

Vegan diets are usually low in fat, helping to reduce the risk of related illnesses like heart disease and obesity. Foods like oil, vegan margarine and nut butters should be used in moderation as they can be high in fat. Olive oil is a good alternative, being rich in mono-unsaturated fats which may reduce the risk of heart disease. However, it should still be taken in moderation; a general guide is one teaspoon per person in a meal.

Iodine

Iodine helps the thyroid gland to work effectively. It can be found in cereals, seaweed and grains.

Iron

Iron is needed for healthy red blood cells. Sources include fortified cereal, wholemeal bread, nuts, leafy green vegetables and pulses. It is easier for the body to absorb plant-based iron if it is taken with food containing vitamin C, e.g. a piece of citrus fruit.

Catherine Greenall

Magnesium

Magnesium helps the parathyroid gland to work and also helps to get energy from food. Sources include bread, nuts, and leafy green vegetables.

Omega Oils and Essential Fatty Acids

Omega oils and essential fatty acids are thought to reduce the risk of heart disease. They can be found in certain vegetable oils, e.g. linseed, rapeseed, flaxseed, walnut and in quinoa.

Phosphorous

Phosphorous is needed for healthy bones and teeth and also helps to get energy from food. Sources include pulses, bread, oats, rice and Brazil nuts.

Potassium

Potassium helps control the fluid balance in the body and may reduce blood pressure. Sources include fruit, especially bananas, wholemeal bread, pulses nuts and seeds.

Protein

Protein is composed of amino acids which are essential for effective functioning of the body's cells and processes. Sources include nuts, seeds, green vegetables, soya products e.g. tofu, cereals and bread.

Selenium

Selenium is important for the functioning of the thyroid, the body's immune system and in reproduction. Sources include Brazil nuts, bread and vegetables.

Vitamin A

Vitamin A is important for healthy skin, the immune system and eyesight. Sources include carrots, orange-coloured fruits, green leafy vegetables and fortified margarines.

B Vitamins

B vitamins are important for energy, functioning of the nervous system, metabolism, heart, healthy skin and blood and energy. Sources include wholegrains, fortified breakfast cereals, nuts and green leafy vegetables.

Vitamin B12

Vitamin B12 is essential for healthy blood and nervous systems. Vegans and vegetarians can be at risk from its deficiency, as it is usually occurs in animal sources. However, it can also be found in fortified breakfast cereals and soya milk.

Vitamin C

Vitamin C is important for healthy tissues, healing and to help the body absorb iron from food. Sources include oranges, sweet potatoes, kiwis and green vegetables.

Vitamin D

Vitamin D is important for healthy bones and to help absorb calcium and phosphorous. It is found in fortified margarines and breakfast cereals. It can also be made in the body by the action of sunlight on the skin.

Vitamin E

Vitamin E is an antioxidant and may protect cells from free radicals, which may lead to cancer, heart and other aging-related illnesses. Sources include green leafy vegetables, nuts, seeds, soya and olive oil.

Vitamin K

Vitamin K is essential for blood clotting and healthy bones. It is found in green leafy vegetables, vegetable oil and cereals.

Zinc

Zinc is important for growth, healing and the reproduction and immune systems. It can be found in cereals, nuts and pulses.

Chapter 6:
References & Further Reading

The Vegan Society	www.vegansociety.com
Why Vegan? The Vegan Society	www.vegansociety.com
The BSE Enquiry	www.bseinquiry.gov.uk
BBC News	www.News.bbc.co.uk
The Daily Mail	www.dailymail.co.uk
Environment, Health & Safety Online	www.ehso.com
Food Standards Agency	www.eatwell.gov.uk
National Health Service	www.5aday.nhs.uk
British Nutrition Foundation	www.nutrition.org.uk
Vegetarian Resource Group	www.vrg.org/index.htm
The Soil Association	www.soilassociation.org
GM Watch	http://www.gmwatch.eu
Wrexham Veggies	http://www.wrexhamveg.org
Vegan Village	http://www.veganvillage.co.uk
Farmers Arms Bispham	http://www.facebook.com/pages/Parbold-United-Kingdom/Farmers-Arms-Bispham-Green/213274616825

Index

Lightning Source UK Ltd.
Milton Keynes UK
02 May 2010

153638UK00001B/13/P